Counterclockwise
Using Peptides to Renew, Rejuvenate, and Rediscover

By Suzanne J Ferree, M.D.,
FAARM, ABAARM

Ghostwriter: Miriam Drennan

Disclaimer

This book contains opinions and ideas, which I have formed and created based on my personal and professional experience treating patients. It is intended to provide helpful general information on the subjects that it addresses. It is not in any way a substitute for the advice of a physician, physicians, or other medical professionals based on one's own individual conditions, symptoms, or concerns. The reader is not to construe or conclude that any medical or other advice is being given concerning the subject matter of the book, and no reader is considered to be a patient as a result of purchasing, using, or reading this book. If the listener needs personal medical health, dietary, exercise, or other assistance or advice, the reader should consult a competent independent physician and you expressly understand that, or other qualified healthcare professionals. The book is not intended, in any form or manner, to be medical advice or substitute advice for consultation with a licensed practitioner. Both myself and those contributing to this book disclaim, all responsibility, liability, damages, or otherwise, at law, in equity, by statute, or in contract, for injury, damage, adverse effects, consequences, or loss that the reader may incur, and any user, purchaser or reader expressly waives any and all claims concerning same, as a direct or indirect consequence of following any information, instructions, directions, preparations, procedures, or suggestions given or discussed in this book, using any products or services described in this book, or participating in any programs mentioned, referenced expressly, or impliedly in this book. I recommend that you consult with your own physician or healthcare specialist regarding the suggestions and recommendations made in this book. The purchase and/or use of this book implies your express consent and acceptance of this disclaimer. The author makes no representations or warranties, express or implied, about the completeness, accuracy, reliability, suitability, or availability with respect to the information, products, services, or related graphics contained in this book for any purpose. Any use of the information is at your own risk.

Dedication

To the only God, our Savior, through Jesus Christ our Lord, be glory, majesty, dominion, and authority, before all time and now and forever. Amen.

Jude 1: 25 (New Revised Standard Version)

Contents

Introduction 5

Chapter 1: Intestinal Health 20

Chapter 2: Immune Function 33

Chapter 3: Energy 46

Chapter 4: Cognitive Issues 58

Chapter 5: Weight Loss 70

Chapter 6: Human Performance 86

Chapter 7: Sleep 103

Chapter 8: Infertility, Perimenopause,
and Other Female-Specific Issues 116

Chapter 9: Skin Care and Hair Loss 139

Conclusion 146

Endnotes 152

INTRODUCTION

"Okay, I'm ready to begin building more muscle," Elizabeth said, greeting me with a smile. "What do we need to do next?"

This was a far cry from the Elizabeth who arrived for her consultation just three short months ago. At fifty-seven, Elizabeth was married, had three adult children, and was a grandmother to one grandchild with another on the way. And she was beyond tired—not the sort of tired someone should feel at fifty-seven.

She had always considered herself to be the type of person who prioritized her health. When she noticed the faint lines forming on her face in her late thirties, she researched ingredients and tried a number of products before coming up with her own skin care formula. She started giving it away as gifts until a friend offered to sell a few jars at her gift shop, which developed into a highly successful business for Elizabeth.

Eventually, she quit her job as a senior accountant to focus squarely on her own small line of healthy, daily-usage products—skin care, coffee, household cleaners—and developed a beloved, trusted brand among those who were like-minded about their health and environment.

By the time she reached her late forties, Elizabeth noticed that it was getting more and more difficult to handle all that she managed. She could still get through her day—working, running kids to football practice and guitar lessons, cooking dinner, helping with yard and house work, volunteering, and church—but by the end of it, she was exhausted. She was even waking up exhausted. She was putting on weight, struggling to remember details that once came easily, forgetting appointments, and even her custom facial cream that started it all for her years ago no longer had the same effect on her skin. Even though she still got in her workouts several times a week, her performance levels were slipping.

When menopause hit a few years later, Elizabeth was reluctant to take estrogen because her doctor would only prescribe a synthetic form of it, and therefore, never did any sort of hormone-replacement therapy. By now, she felt clumsy and old, and was appreciative of the company of her golden doodles and husband. Watching her children leave the nest one-by-one left her wondering what to do with the extra time on her hands. She didn't have to wait long.

Her mother fell and broke her hip, leaving her unable to care for Elizabeth's father, who had dementia. His caretaking fell to Elizabeth, who struggled to take on the role in her exhausted state. Though he recognized his daughter most days, Elizabeth's father would get agitated with her when he didn't understand why he couldn't drive his car or help her with her mother. Emotional stress compounded her fatigue.

"I'm barely checking the boxes," she said to me at her first appointment. "But I also know that's a lot of boxes for anyone to check at my age."

Frankly, it was a lot of boxes at *any* age. Yet Elizabeth was open to something more, something different. Something beyond her primary care physician telling her she needed to accept that she was merely aging.

"I'm not trying to be a supermodel or anything like that," she told me. "I just want to feel like myself again. As active as I've been all my life, I feel like my energy and stamina have taken a nosedive, and that can't be normal. I don't even recognize the person in the mirror anymore. I'm in there . . . somewhere."

I knew I could help her, at least where her allopathic doctor couldn't.

The first thing we did was talk about her lifestyle modification. She was doing a lot of cardio exercise, but we needed to begin working on resistance exercise, which is important to add as we age. As my friend and health and wellness podcaster, Carl Lanore says, "Muscle is the currency of aging, so get in the gym and make a deposit today."

We also went through her diet with a fine-tooth comb and adjusted her macros, which are the percentage of protein, carbohydrate, and fat that made up her daily diet. Once we had this foundation, we began adding in anti-aging supplements and peptides to address cellular aging and immunosenescence, the aging of the immune system. She took treatments for skin aging and arthritis prevention, some of which were injectable into the muscle and joints. Because of these injections, she was able to resolve a knee problem without surgery.

It's not just Elizabeth who is living proof of peptide therapy's real impact. I was able to help a client with a meniscus tear return to her favorite sport without resorting to surgery. For yet another client, peptide therapy prevented her requiring a hip replacement for avascular necrosis—and now, she's back to doing CrossFit.

This is the power of individualized, patient-focused cellular medicine. To develop a treatment plan for my clients, we start by doing an intricately detailed health history, which includes dental and dietary health, potential toxin exposures (such as water- damaged buildings and plastic food containers), and any past concussions. Then, we do a large panel of blood work to determine what we need to add or modify in the patient's peptide stack, their unique combination of peptides. There's a plan from day one, and it's constantly refined to best meet the client's shifting needs and goals.

Understanding the way peptides work at the cellular level is critical. This is part of why you shouldn't purchase them from a research lab and do it yourself; if you don't understand how they work at the cellular level, you may not be able to properly combine or use them so that you get the best result.

If you're like Elizabeth, you have too much going on . . . in a good way. To have enough energy for all of it, you want to stay as young as you can for as long as you can. You want a treatment plan that works *with* you, not just for you.

If You Could Turn Back Time

Everyone ages. It's a part of life. The fatigue that prevents you from doing everything you want or should be able to do. The difficulty of losing weight, despite exercise and diet. Poor sleep, low libido, lackluster hair and skin . . .

 . . . poor memory, brain fog, sluggish cognitive function and executive function, difficulty finding words, an inability to concentrate and focus, (did I mention poor memory?) . . .

 . . . not recovering from workouts, feeling sore days after exercising, losing your competitive athletic edge . . .

Should I keep going, or do you recognize yourself in these symptoms? Aging doesn't have to feel like this.

At what age did you last feel like the best, most energized version of yourself? What if I told you that you could feel like that again without a time machine?

Peptide therapy might sound like magic, but trust me: there is a lot of scientific support for its miraculous benefits. Before we get into how we can make peptides work for you, let's start with a crash course in what peptides are so we can understand how they impact our health.

A Brief Lesson in Peptides

There are thousands and thousands of peptides in our body, each with its own specialized job. They are essential in helping our body function, but their importance wasn't known until the 1920s. Dr. Ivan Pavlov—yes, as in the doctor who did the famous behavioral conditioning experiment with the dogs—discovered that nervous signals control digestion. Originally, he studied the function of dogs' intestines, and based on his research, other scientists stumbled upon secretin, which is a peptide involved in digestive health.

This breakthrough opened the floodgates into peptide research. Several more peptides were discovered in quick succession. One of these peptides is insulin, which is probably the peptide most people are familiar with even if they don't realize that it's a peptide. Other common peptides include bacitracin, which is a topical antibiotic, and the blood pressure medicine losartan.

Peptides are everywhere. We just don't know them as peptides. Every time your body requires an enzyme to do a job, it has to make a peptide to make that happen. Peptides and proteins are both made of amino acids. A protein is greater than 150 amino acids in length, and a peptide is less than fifty amino acids in length. A polypeptide is between 50 and 150 amino acids in length. Your body takes the proteins that you eat and breaks them down into tiny little amino acids. These amino acids are the body's building blocks that are structured into the proteins and peptides it needs to do its job.

Since 2005, we have been able to create these in a lab. Until then, we had to obtain these proteins from an animal or from another human. We still use these natural sources to some degree, such as an insulin called NPH that is acquired from pigs. Peptides used to be synthesized on a solid support by hand in a process called *solid-phase synthesis*. Using solid-phase synthesis, getting these peptides was so labor-, time-, and resource-intensive that we weren't able to make them in a way that was commercially reasonable. Now, we can create peptides in a lab with a peptide synthesizer and manufacture these series of amino acids into the peptides that we want in large enough quantities that they can be used commercially.

Another benefit of lab-produced peptides is that we are able to replicate the exact sequence of amino acids that your body naturally makes. When they derive from an animal source, the sequence of amino acids is going to be slightly different than what a human naturally produces. Because of this difference, it might not do the exact same thing as the human amino acids. Lab-produced amino acids are bioidentical even though they're synthetic, and in this way, they're familiar to your body. Your body senses them as itself and is able to fully put them to use.

Why Are Peptides Important?

As we age, *how* our body uses these amino acids changes. When a twenty-year-old eats a chicken breast, those proteins are broken down into its amino acids, which absorbed into her intestine. The cells of her body take those amino acids and make the new proteins and peptides her body needs, especially for all of the reproductive processes a twenty-year-old's body needs to fuel. As we age, our body tries to conserve energy. It begins to fold up the pieces of the DNA blueprint that are involved in more youthful processes like collagen for the skin and reproduction. When that twenty-year-old is eighty, there's no need for her body to make those reproductive proteins. These blueprints are wrapped up on spools called *histones*, which become inaccessible to prevent the unnecessary energy expenditure of making those particular proteins.

Youthful proteins are depleted, such as the ones that come from the thymus gland and are involved in the immune system vitality. The reason why elderly patients are more susceptible to illnesses such as COVID is because their bodies aren't spending as much energy creating all of the peptides needed to strengthen their immune system.

The bad news is this process happens much earlier than eighty. We have a system that is designed to start aging about thirty-five years old. Around this age, we decrease our production of immune system and reproductive hormones, proteins, and peptides. As we age, we are conserving more and more energy. I can feed an eighty-year-old as much protein as I want, but I'm not going to get the more youthful expression of their DNA unless I use GHK or Thymosin Alpha-1 or BPC peptides that help unwind that shelved DNA from its spools and allow their production.

Peptide Therapy

So how do we get these peptides from the lab into the client? It all starts in the lab, where the peptide is made. These labs are FDA-approved, which means they monitor the machines and product for their sterility and quality. Then the peptide is sent to a compounding pharmacy, where it's packaged and sent out after ensuring it has at least 99 percent purity of exactly what protein we want and no infections. These are then sent to the patient or to the doctor's office in a vial, where they are administered subcutaneously as an injection that goes just under the skin, into a tendon or joint, or administered through an IV.

Because nobody likes a shot, new technologies are rapidly developing for other delivery methods. Some peptides are available orally, intranasally, or through a topical cream or transdermal patch. This science is evolving every day, but for now, most of them are only available by injection.

A lot of the topicals and orals are available over the counter, but they are not going to give you the efficacy that you want for systemic problems, which would benefit the most from injections. A topical cream might penetrate one or two layers of skin, but it won't reach the parts you need to target for an immune system challenge. If you want to get these peptides to your heart muscle, liver muscle, or brain, an injection is the best way to ensure the amount you need is going where they are needed most.

While there are plenty of online sources for peptides, these are not meant for human consumption. These are research labs that make peptides for animal research, and as such, they don't have the rigorous testing needed for human medicine. Compounding pharmacies are required to go through third-party testing in order to administer these treatments safely to humans.

Why is Peptide Therapy Not a Fad?

Unlike health fads, like diet pills and "healthy" smoking, peptide therapy isn't a trend that we will look back on with humor and a twinge of regret. There are thousands of articles supporting the use of these peptides, some dating back to the 1920s when secretin was first identified. New peptides are identified all the time—and they are doing amazing things in our bodies. Because this research is rapidly developing, it requires constant vigilance on the part of medical practitioners to stay ahead of the curve on what is available. I have devoted my career to peptide research, and I'm still surprised every day. I find new things all the time, and I'm constantly figuring out how I can incorporate them into my clients' treatment to help them feel the best they can.

Controversy

In January 2024, the Food and Drug Administration (FDA) released a list of peptides they want to ban compounding pharmacies from being able to make for our patients. This proposed ban includes many of the peptides we commonly and safely use with excellent outcomes for our patients. The proposed ban is not due to peptides causing any illness or deaths in patients using peptides from compounding pharmacies. The only reported serious adverse events (SAEs) in patients have been in those obtaining peptides from black market sources. While I have some conjecture as to the cause of this proposed ban, I can only encourage you that we are working with lawyers to restrain the FDA from this proposed ban. We are also working with compounding pharmacies to discover effective alternative peptides to take care of our patients. My next book will include these alternatives and more discoveries!

Looking Ahead

I know you probably haven't heard many doctors say this, but I love it when patients do their own research. There is so much information out there that I cannot keep up with it all by myself. When patients bring me research, it's very exciting. If, however, you're a little overwhelmed, I get it. This is a lot of science, but this book won't make you feel like you are in chemistry class.

Using this book as a tool, you will be able to take this knowledge and advocate for your own peptide treatment plan with your doctor. Or, you'll be able to ask your doctor to turn to me to learn how to create these peptide combinations. I have provided references in the form of a PubMed ID number (PMID) to help you find the specific article that I reference.

Seeking Treatment

The reality is that science and manufacturers are moving faster than doctors can keep up with. Your primary care doctor is seeing thirty to forty patients a day and is not necessarily going to be well versed in something like peptide treatment unless they have specifically gone back to school to learn about it.

Your general practitioner is probably an allopathic doctor, which means that they treat the symptom, not the cause. If you come to them with high blood pressure, they're going to give you a prescription for your high blood pressure. If you come to them for your headache, they're going to give you a prescription for your headache. The root problem is still there, just masked. The medication is intended to address the specific symptom, regardless of side effects—or, sometimes, additional benefits. This is how allopathic doctors are trained, this is the work they do, and we encourage our patients to maintain that very important relationship they have with their primary care provider.

Cellular medicine providers have a different approach. Our goal is to figure out *why* your cells are creating high blood pressure and headache. We ask how we can reset the nerves, muscle cells, and heart cells so that they are able to do their optimal work. Cellular medicine providers treat the cause, not the symptom. Instead of simply managing the high blood pressure or headache, we work to eliminate it.

Some, but not all, allopathic practitioners are not open to the idea of cellular medicine and, subsequently, peptide therapy, usually because they haven't done the research or haven't been exposed to it. With medicine in general, the world of insurance has restricted allopathic doctors to believe that there isn't anything out there besides what the drug reps tell them. Usually, their biggest source of information comes from these salesmen because that's the only thing they have time for.

To some degree, medical school education is supported by the drug companies. Unless your doctor is really curious, there's not a lot of time or room for questions. Medical school tends to crush an allopathic doctor's curiosity out of them, instructing that there is one way to do things. They learn the one way to do it, they follow that prescription, and then they don't really deviate from that until the drug rep brings them a new drug to use as a tool.

Because there is an overwhelming number of new drugs constantly hitting the market, doctors struggle to keep up with what all those drugs do beyond what the drug rep says; many are not giving the patient the best possible care they can have. A cellular medicine doctor's practice is based on curiosity; when presented with a new drug, they ask what the mechanism of action is, and then do all the research they can.

For example, the popular diabetes medication that's often prescribed for weight loss is a peptide. If you have not done the research, it's easy to assume that it is only for diabetes and weight loss. Originally, this drug was researched for patients with dementia and Parkinson's. It had some good outcomes, but the patients lost too much weight—and those are usually thin patients already. Someone realized they could capitalize on the side effect and formulate it for diabetes and weight loss.

Unfortunately, with a lot of the research that is available right now, the goal is to get drugs into the hands of the pharmaceutical company so that they can make money. There's not a lot of capital gain in a natural, un-synthesized product, because it can't be patented. So the cycle continues: development, drug rep, prescription, treatment of symptom. Lather, rinse, repeat.

I understand the doubts of many allopathic doctors when it comes to peptide therapy. With any cutting-edge medicine, there's always fear around trying things with patients because some treatments are not FDA-approved and, as a doctor, you don't want to risk your license. Our cardinal rule of medicine is to do no harm. There is always a concern that I might be hurting my patient by prescribing something the FDA hasn't fully approved, which is why I am so dedicated to research and finding the best—and safest—solution for my clients.

My Background

I went to medical school at Eastern Virginia Medical School in Norfolk, Virginia, where I did some infertility research. Then I moved to Atlanta and went to Emory for residency and family medicine, thinking I was going to be a regular doctor working for a big, insurance-based company. Every day, I would walk in at eight o'clock in the morning and go home at seven. If a patient came in with a symptom, I had a drug for every disease. But as I went along, I realized that I didn't have a drug for every disease. Maybe that lens actually wasn't the way to think about treatment. Instead, maybe I should help them optimize the way all of their cells work as early as I can, and possibly intervene so that those symptoms don't arise in the first place.

A new drug might have benefited five of my four-thousand patients, but I still had that many patients who had some sort of illness I wanted to address. I started looking into natural therapies at the request of my patients, who asked me about remedies such as saw palmetto. I didn't know what that was, so I looked it up. This was back in the 1990s, so the Google search didn't exist like it does now. I did as much research as I could and if the data suggested the treatment wouldn't hurt, we gave it a try. In this way, my approach was, and still is, very patient-directed. After all, the patient is the one who knows how they feel, so why aren't we listening to them?

They would come back weeks later and say, "Wow, I noticed that my hair isn't falling out like it used to! I feel more energized!" So I started exploring what natural herbal options were available that patients could get over the counter.

As a Navy Lieutenant, I served as the physical fitness coordinator at a military base, which means I helped my military patients pass their physical fitness tests. I brought this knowledge of diet and exercise into my treatment and suggested little things, such as cutting out salty food and increasing exercise to lower blood pressure. A good number of my patients got better with those lifestyle modifications as well as the natural interventions.

Then a patient came to me and said, "Hey, will you fill my prescription for bioidentical hormones?" I didn't know what that was, so I just copied the prescription from the bottle and sent it to the compounding pharmacy, which I had never heard of or engaged with before. The kind compounding pharmacist called me up and said, "Hey, I see that you don't know what you're doing. Can I send you to a conference?"

And so, he did. I went to a medical conference and learned about bioidentical hormones, and it was an awakening. I realized there was a whole world of treatment options that I hadn't known existed. That conference sparked a hunger for more education, and I took as many classes as I possibly could. I did a fellowship program through A4M, the American Academy of Anti-Aging in Regenerative Medicine. This program was about a two-year, mostly remote, intensive functional medicine course. It was very evidence-based, meaning the lecturers are required to use the most research available to teach their subject. It was amazing to me how much research was out there about bioidentical hormones, and that's what started me on the path of cellular medicine. Once I started implementing bioidentical hormones, I saw a lot more of my patients improve and knew that I was on the right track.

Introduction

It wasn't until I injured myself, however, that I discovered peptide therapy. I wasn't a superstar runner, but running was a big part of my life. I competed in some local 5K and 10K races, and everything was going great. That is, until the ages of thirty-five to forty, when I started having hip pain that just wouldn't go away. I tried many different treatments and modalities: dry needling, ultrasound therapy, massage, chiropractic, and physical therapy. But no matter what, I couldn't get better.

I was running an annual 10K race in Atlanta called the Peachtree Road Race, when I had to stop in the middle because it was too painful to continue running. And that was my last race, because I didn't know what else to try.

I went to the annual convention for A4M, and one of the lectures happened to be on a peptide for athletic injury. It was Divine timing. During these lectures, I usually have a pad of paper by my side with a list of patient names. As soon as I hear something that a patient might benefit from, I make note of it by their name. I walked away with a list of peptide treatments to call my patients about, and I made note of what could help me as well. After the lecture, I took a weekend introduction to peptides course and followed that up with the fellowship on peptides through A4M. I started using peptides in my practice every day.

The results were immediate. I saw a return to sport quicker than expected and an improvement in recovery time. Clients are able to exercise more days in a week, have increased muscle mass gain, improved fat loss, improved cognition in patients with mild cognitive impairment, improved sleep quality, resolution of longstanding intestinal problems, resolution of arthritic pain and tendinopathies, improved markers of aging, and shortened courses of illnesses, like COVID.

Now, I'm using a combination of natural remedies, lifestyle modifications, bioidentical hormones, and peptide therapy that has created amazing results for the health and wellness of my patients . . . and even myself. Once I started using peptides, my hip no longer bothers me, although I am a competitive powerlifter, and many patients who previously stayed sick with an allopathic approach recovered under my care.

I've experienced the success of peptide treatment firsthand, and I want more people who were previously hopeless about their stubborn health issues to experience its benefits.

What This Book Is and Isn't

This book is a comprehensive review of the available peptides for enhancing health and function. To a certain extent, this book will be an introduction to cellular health. Along those same lines, it will demonstrate how cellular health is connected to longevity.

This book is not, however, suggesting that peptide therapy is the panacea. The patient has a proactive role in their health that includes careful attention to diet, exercise, sleep habits, stress management, and so on. Peptide therapy assists, but it should not be considered a form of cure-all magic.

As you read, keep in mind that peptide therapy is used in conjunction with the other treatments and modifications. Those things need to be in place in order for peptides to be effective.

Each chapter is categorized based on groups of peptides, what they treat, and how they work. Note that there will be a lot of overlap, because a cell is a cell is a cell. If I'm fixing one kind of cell, I'm probably fixing other kinds of cells. This book is designed so that you can either read it cover-to-cover or skip to the sections that apply to you.

The chapters will be body-area focused, with examples from my own patients and some physiology and biochemistry that you can read or skip through. Each chapter will also have a deeper dive on a particular topic that's relative to the chapter.

First Things First: The Gut Feeling

Although this is designed to be a skip-around reference book, I encourage you to read Chapter One, as intestinal health is the base of all our health. It can trigger all kinds of health problems that might not be obvious at first, so let's get into the importance of the 'gut feeling' on the rest of our health.

CHAPTER ONE

Intestinal Health

Elle was a sixty-year-old executive who had enjoyed a very active lifestyle and ran a very successful business. She cares for her elderly mother, whom she moved into her home a few years prior, and loves caring for her four young granddaughters a few days each week.

Even though she was happily remarried following a traumatic divorce several years prior, Elle retained the trauma of her previous marriage that left her with some fairly significant PTSD. This manifested as intestinal symptoms: debilitating diarrhea, significant weight loss, and so on. Though she has a family history of Crohn's disease and many of her symptoms were similar, thus far it had not been found in her.

The diarrhea and weight loss begin to affect her ability to function in the boardroom, in the weight room, at her home, and in the bedroom. "I can't go on like this," she told me tearfully. "What is happening to me?"

The Source of All Illness?

For many years, allopathic and even functional medicine doctors did not hear their naturopathic colleagues telling them that the large and small intestines are the source of all illness. The immune system lives just inside the intestinal wall, only one cell layer between the outside world and the inside; it's parked there, like a centurion, just waiting for the entry of an invader.

What sort of invaders are we talking about? It varies from person to person, but certainly gluten, stress, or infections—like bacteria or viruses—can cause the breakdown of that one cell layer. Once it allows entry of food particles and infections into the body, this triggers the immune response. An activated immune system will wreak havoc all over the body, causing things like skin rashes, brain fog, heart problems, and liver malfunction, just to name a few.

As you navigate through your health journey, keep this in mind: *If your intestines are working the way they are supposed to, everything else falls into place.*

Therefore, a raised awareness of symptoms that indicate something is out of whack is required. For instance, you should be moving your bowels at least once a day, and it should be easy to pass. Children's bowels move after just about every meal, and it's fantastic if you can move them as often as an adult. Regardless, you shouldn't have to stress or strain to move them.

If you're doing anything less than one easy pass per day, then it's probably a little bit of constipation. If you're passing very loose, more liquid than solid stools, it's diarrhea. If those bowels are watery, not only does this suggest infection, but you can also easily become dehydrated.

Another ailment directly linked to intestinal health is increased intestinal permeability, commonly known as "leaky gut syndrome." Remember, only one cell layer stands between the world and your body—the intestinal epithelial cells. That cell layer is the gatekeeper, and it can be breached by things like gluten, stress, viruses, and bacteria. Once breached, other things can get into the body that aren't supposed to get into the body. The immune system then attacks what should just be amino acids and vitamins that have already been digested, but because of the breakdown of the intestinal epithelial layer, these things can "leak" in and gain access to our immune system, which immediately creates an antibody to what it perceives as an invader. As a result, we've created allergies and food sensitivities.

This is more than just diarrhea, constipation, and leaky gut, however; smaller things, like bloating after eating a particular food or experiencing heartburn or reflux, need more than a cursory acknowledgement. These not only indicate that you may not digest certain foods well, but they also are giving advance warning about your immune system before more severe complications occur. Those random moments, where you just feel kind of "off," should not be dismissed either—they could be an early indicator that is linked to your intestinal health, too.

What's Happening at the Cellular Level

One of the coolest concepts to grasp here is the way that intestinal cells work. There is this beautiful, symbiotic relationship between the healthy bugs that live in your gut and the intestinal epithelial cells—that one-cell layer thick between the world and your body that I mentioned earlier. This beautiful relationship is recognized when you eat fiber; it goes into your intestines. Your happy, healthy intestinal bugs will eat that fiber and convert it into your intestinal epithelial cells' preferred fuel source called butyrate. This is a fat that gives those cells all the energy they need.

Just like the other cells in your body, those cells have the option to choose which foods they prefer; kind of like when we're trying to decide what to eat and we have the choice of eating Twizzlers, a chicken breast, a baked potato, and so on. The cells have the choice of sugar without oxygen, sugar with oxygen, fat, or protein.

- Sugar without oxygen produces about two packets of energy (called ATP).
- Sugar with oxygen produces about thirty packets of energy.

- Fat, used as a substitute for sugar, produces about a hundred packages of energy.
- Protein breakdown is undesirable, as it comes primarily from muscle. Muscle is the source of many anti-inflammatory signaling chemicals and what keeps us upright, doing the things we love. We don't want our cells using this source if at all possible.

It's clear that fat is the most efficient energy source, and the cell functions optimally when it has plenty of energy.

Bottom line: a happy intestinal epithelial cell, a happy brain cell, a happy heart muscle cell, or a happy liver cell all function optimally when they have as much energy as they need in order to accomplish their job for the day. By the same token, bugs in the intestine digest fiber from your diet and create delicious butyrate for your intestinal epithelial cells. Those cells then take that fat and make a hundred packets of energy. They suck up all the oxygen from the bloodstream, leaving the intestinal lumen an oxygen-less or hypoxic space perfect for the "good bugs" that function well without oxygen. The good bugs love to be in an hypoxic environment that gives all the energy-making resources to your intestinal epithelial cells. In turn, the intestinal epithelial cells aren't panicking, because they have all the nutrients, all the oxygen, everything they need. This is a beautiful, symbiotic relationship.

If you have a colonoscopy prep, three days of antibiotics, or a stomach flu, this erases those 'good bugs' from the lumen and the 'bad bugs' take over, stealing all the oxygen so your intestinal epithelial cells (IECs) can't make the energy they need. Stressed cells may ultimately result in diseases like ulcerative colitis or colon cancer.

Individual Peptides

Peptides are strings of fewer than fifty amino acids with a signaling function within or between cells. As I mentioned in the Introduction, most peptides are known by numerical and alphabet letter names because they are not owned by a pharmaceutical company yet (familiar exceptions to this are the peptides Bacitracin, a topical antibiotic and Losartan, an oral blood pressure medicine). Peptides work synergistically with your intestinal epithelial cells.

If you take an antibiotic, prepare for colonoscopy, or have an intestinal bug like a viral gastroenteritis or stomach flu, all of a sudden you have completely changed your microbiome and allowed for the overgrowth of bugs that like to be in an oxygenated environment. Now your intestinal epithelial cells are competing with the microbes in your intestines for oxygen; if they don't have enough oxygen to make the energy they need, your intestinal epithelial cells begin to participate in the inflammatory response. Working in tandem with lifestyle changes, dietary changes, and supplements, peptides can be the final push that rights the ship.

When it comes to intestinal health, I commonly prescribe for my patients any of the following peptides:

BPC-157

This is a fifteen-amino acid fragment of the naturally occurring body protection compound that comes from your stomach. It was first discovered in 1990 as a crucial mediator of the stomach stress-coping response.

While most peptides are available by injection, BPC-157 is also available orally because the original peptide from which it was taken is an intestinal peptide from the stomach. It can actually tolerate the very, very low and acidic pH of the stomach.[1]

BPC-157 is a membrane stabilizer and treats leaky gut by improving capillary permeability (i.e., the blood flow to the area). [2] It also protects organs outside the intestinal tract, like the endothelium, which is the lining of the blood vessels. Because of its effect on many receptors in the body on different cells, it has tremendous anti-inflammatory effects; BPC-157 even has effects on the dopamine and serotonin systems in the brain, which influence mood and energy.[3]

It decreases ulcers of the stomach and duodenum, which is the first part of the small intestine, after stress exposure. Researchers exposed rats, mice, and chickens to heat-cold, restraint, alcohol, and acid; the animals developed ulcers in their stomach as a result. When they were pretreated with BPC-157, however, subjects did not develop ulcers.[4]

One of the problems with reflux or heartburn is that the tight band at the bottom of the esophagus—located between the esophagus and the stomach—relaxes, allowing acid to reflux back up into the esophagus. The esophagus isn't supposed to see any acid, and when it does, patients may experience the symptoms of reflux. Anti-inflammatories (like ibuprofen), stress, large meals, caffeine, and nicotine can also cause relaxation of that lower esophageal sphincter. In a separate trial, rats were given an anti-inflammatory drug, which caused relaxation of the lower esophageal sphincter. When given BPC-157, each one's lower esophageal sphincter function was restored.[5]

While the focus of this chapter is intestinal health, BPC-157 has also benefited subjects with osteoarthritis, Parkinson's Disease, and spinal cord injury. This peptide is amazing!

Vasoactive Intestinal Peptide (VIP)

VIP is a twenty-eight amino acid neuropeptide that was isolated from the small intestine of pigs in 1970. It's produced by neurons in the brain, nerve cells, and immune cells, but it's present in most of the organs of the body. It regulates hormone secretion and motility of the intestinal tract; that's how it functions in the intestine, regulating insulin and other hormone releases for metabolic function.

In one study, VIP reduced the clinical severity of Crohn's disease, including weight loss, diarrhea, and macroscopic inflammation. Examining intestinal specimens under the microscope, researchers saw that they had a significant decrease in their inflammation. They also looked at the chemical messengers of inflammation, like tumor necrosis factor alpha (TNF-alpha) and IL-6, and discovered they had decreased, resulting in a reduced food allergy response.[6]

Ipamorelin

Ipamorelin is a growth-hormone secretagogue, which means it increases the release of growth hormone from the pituitary. Using Ipamorelin, patients won't overdose on growth hormone because they're not receiving actual growth hormone; instead, they receive something that's going to encourage the secretion of their own growth hormone.

The best thing about Ipamorelin is that it will release growth hormone within a respectable high potency and effectiveness, but it doesn't increase stress hormone levels, which growth hormone itself would increase.

Ipamorelin has benefited postoperative cases where the intestines are very slow to respond; it increases stool frequency, food intake, and restores body weight after surgery. There are several studies showing that—for patients who struggle with constipation—ipamorelin is a great way to improve the way the intestinal epithelial cells choose to use energy.[7]

AT-1001

AT-1001 is an oral peptide that is locally active in the intestines. It is a tight junction regulator. Remember those intestinal epithelial cells? They have small gates between them, like fences between houses in a neighborhood; these are called tight junctions and, in good health, they are selectively permeable. Remember that behind the intestinal epithelial cells sits the immune system. If that tight junction or that gate is broken down, then things can get into the body that aren't supposed to, like bacteria, viruses, and broccoli. AT-1001 regulates that barrier, and prevents it from opening, which blocks things from reaching your intestinal immunity and triggering this inflammatory response. It improves leaky gut or intestinal permeability, and is specifically being studied in patients with celiac disease.[8]

In fact, patients who took this and then consumed gluten, AT-1001 prevented their gluten-induced symptoms. It decreased their antibody production, improved their leaky gut, and prevented the production of all the inflammatory chemicals with a safety profile that was comparable to placebo.[9]

There is also evidence that indicates AT-1001 works against COVID-19, which is awesome.[10] The interesting thing about AT-1001 is that you will know within two weeks if your body will respond well to it; patients should expect to see significant improvement in their skin and intestinal symptoms.

LL37

LL37 is a thirty-seven amino acid, positively charged, antimicrobial peptide that is produced by the colon cells. And I have to admit, I think it's so cool that our colon cells make their own antimicrobials!

Then, someone who was really smart found it and said, "Oh, we can make this in a lab. If someone's intestines aren't working properly, we can actually give them this so that they can have an antibacterial or antimicrobial effect!" LL37 penetrates the bacterial membrane and forms pores in the cell wall so that the bacteria cannot survive.

When bacteria invade your body, they produce a film that lays over them that is created by other bacteria, yeast, and other things to hide from your immune system. We call that a biofilm. A biofilm is protective of the dominant bacteria or dominant virus, hiding it from your immune system by covering itself in this blanket of schmutz—mucus, other bugs, and immune cells that either tried to help and got killed in the process or are symbiotic (meaning they benefit from association with the primary microbe).

LL37 reduces the biofilm so that now your immune system can actually see the bugs that are there, including the dominant bug; you can actually recruit your immune system to kill it rather than be distracted by all the schmutz. It is effective against all kinds of pathogens!

This little peptide can be effective against bacteria; viruses like herpes and rhinovirus (common cold); Borrelia, which causes Lyme disease; lots of intestinal bugs, like Klebsiella and E. coli.[11] That said, proceed with caution: when used in excess, LL37 can act as an antigen and assist a flare-up of psoriasis when psoriasis is already present in the body. So if you already have psoriasis, I would not recommend using LL37.

Peptide Stacks

There are thousands of peptides working every day in your body, doing their jobs all together at the same time. When we prescribe peptides for our patients, we often will provide them in "stacks," or combinations of multiple peptides—usually, anywhere from two to five, depending on the circumstances. An anti-aging stack would look different than an intestinal health stack; an intestinal health stack would look different in someone with Crohn's disease than in someone with stomach ulcerations. Peptide stacks are based on your baseline health, how they work in your body, and what we know about the disease state, if there is one present.

For example, if someone suffers from intestinal ailments, like acid reflux disease, we would begin by thoroughly reviewing and implementing any lifestyle changes—how are they managing stress, how much fiber is in their diet, are they drinking too much coffee or too much alcohol, are they "eating" ibuprofen, and so on. We would also coordinate with their primary care provider to ensure our course of treatment complements any other strategies that are in place for the patient. I would probably start them with two double doses of BPC-157 per day; they would open one capsule and pour the contents in water and take with another capsule that is still intact.

In many cases, these patients take proton pump inhibitors (PPIs), like omeprazole, and this regimen can help them to gradually wean off them, as chronic PPI use has been associated with the development of osteoporosis and recurrent infections. If their symptoms are stress-induced, I would add AT-1001, having them take it at least once a day before their heaviest meal or a meal that might include wheat (even though my preference would be that they give up wheat altogether). So if they typically don't have pasta for dinner, but always have a croissant for breakfast, then they would want to take it before the croissant. But if they always have pasta for dinner, then they would want to take it before the pasta.

If a patient came in with Crohn's disease, I would probably add VIP to that regimen, as long as they weren't having diarrhea—VIP moves the bowels along pretty quickly—and Thymus Alpha 1, which is a peptide we'll dig into in the next chapter. If they were having diarrhea, I might use a GLP-1 peptide called semaglutide. A standard leaky gut protocol would probably include VIP, AT-1001, and a third peptide called KPV, which is anti-inflammatory that we'll also discuss more in-depth in the next chapter.

These peptides work in slightly different ways, but they all work at the cellular level. We use them together to optimize and synergize the effects. Stacking them in this way gives you far more benefits than taking a single one by itself. Think about it like this: you could eat a chicken breast for dinner and get some nutrients that way, but if you had one that's Parmesan-encrusted, and came with roasted asparagus and mushrooms with créme fraîche, that meal would give you all the nutrients that you might need (not to mention a delicious taste!).

The peptides are only a contributor to the solution, however. Treating the intestines includes a lot of dietary changes and natural supplement treatment, like collagen, glutamine, marshmallow, and slippery elm. Peptides are part of the solution, not the solution itself. The impact gut health has on other body systems cannot be ignored, either. Anytime we see someone who has depression, dementia, skin rashes, and heart issues, among others, we are always going to look at what is happening with their intestines first. Nothing is going to get better if we're not starting there.

Final Thoughts

Peptide therapy is not a magic cure-all, and patients must remain active participants in their health journey. There may be dietary and lifestyle changes, or supplements that need to be taken. If I'm treating someone with peptides, the strategy is not turnkey; many who are used to allopathic practitioners may think you visit a functional medicine doctor, they write you a prescription for the peptide, and you move on with your life. In fact, there are several steps we take to ensure optimal results, including discussing any lifestyle changes that may need to be employed, coordinating with their primary care provider or specialists, and so on.

In Elle's case, we discovered she had a food allergy. She was treated with an elimination diet and repair supplements, plus BPC-157 (one open 500 milligram (mg) capsule in water, taken with one 500 mg capsule intact). We resolved her diarrhea, she returned to her baseline weight, and she began to build muscle mass again. Today, she has a beautifully sculpted body and the energy to launch and sustain a new company . . . and still has energy left to keep going!

If you and your provider don't pay attention to your intestinal health, you will increase your chances of developing an autoimmune disease. Increased intestinal permeability exposes us to things not usually seen by the immune system. Because the immune system should only see the outside of that cell or the breakdown products of broccoli, for example, the permeability of the intestines gives the immune system access, and therefore, now sees that cell or food fragment as a foreign entity. Exposure to the outside environment is due to increased intestinal permeability from stress or infections, exposing us to things we aren't always aware of. If your intestinal health is problematic, your immune system may create an antibody to what it considers an invader.

A Closer Look at Leaky Gut

There is pathophysiology of antibiotics and other things that create leaky gut. Your intestinal epithelial cells recruit the immune system to help them fight off this threat; they're telling your immune system, "Hey, I'm stressed out. I need some help."

The stress doesn't always come from antibiotics; it can be a change in your diet, like keto, which has very low carbohydrates and fiber. Your cells can even get stressed just prepping for a colonoscopy. These destroy your microbiome and your intestines.

The healthy bugs in the lumen of your intestines take the fiber in your diet and convert it to butyrate, your intestinal epithelial cells' favorite fatty food. Butyrate provides them with plenty of energy to do their job of water balance, creation of the mucus layer, and production of antimicrobial peptides. When they don't have this energy source, either due to dietary restriction of fiber or due to destruction of healthy bugs by antibiotics, colonoscopy prep, stress, or the stomach flu, intestinal epithelial cells begin to go through a cell danger response.

This may result in damage to the intestinal epithelial cells and disease states like Crohn's, ulcerative colitis, and even colon cancer. One simple way to fix this is by increasing the amount of fiber in your diet so that you're feeding your good bugs, and they're making your intestines their favorite food. Taking a quality probiotic may help in the short-term to replace those lost by poor diet or antibiotic therapy, etc.

There are many books and even more opinions about this; simply put, knowing specific amounts of what your epithelial intestinal cells need is highly individualized, which makes it more difficult. Sometimes, you have to take the butyrate directly; since this fat is the preferred source for colon cells, administering butyrate rectally can be highly effective, as it provides your body and good bacteria with energy. The exact dose would likely need to be sent to a compounding pharmacy.

A liquid form of butyrate is available through a company called KetoneAid, sold as Ke4. A capsule called Tributyrin is also available, and finally, butyrate can be administered orally, intravenously, or per rectum, as sodium butyrate.

Fermented foods contain a lot of healthy bacteria. Foods like kimchi, yogurt, and sauerkraut are all good sources. Sauerkraut, in particular, actually contains glutamine, which also can help restore the mucosal layer on the inside of your intestinal epithelial cells—just one more barrier to protect you.

With leaky gut, the problem is not the overgrowth of bad bacteria; the problem is a stressed out intestinal epithelial cell that doesn't have the ability to make the energy it needs to perform its job. It's competing with not only the bad bacteria in your gut, but also with the immune system for energy resources that are dwindling because of the presence of the bad bacteria.

If you elect to visit a functional medicine doctor, ask them, "What is your protocol for treating leaky gut?" This is a great question because if they don't agree or believe that leaky gut actually exists, that's a doctor you probably should stay away from.

Instead, look for doctors that mention things like slippery elm, marshmallow root, and glutamine, as those are all supplements with evidence-based research backing their use in repairing the mucosal lining as well as the intestinal barrier, which maintains gut integrity.

Finally, if their answer is to take omeprazole or famotidine, then that's a doctor you may want to avoid, and seek additional care from a functional medicine doctor.

CHAPTER TWO

Immune Function

Jane was a sixty-three-year-old married entrepreneur contractor for classified military operations. She and her husband had one adult child, who was about to be married herself. They lived comfortably and were planning a big affair for the wedding. Jane and her girlfriends traveled extensively three or four times per year, stayed in the best hotels, and ate the finest cuisine. She was always well-dressed in boutique clothing and spent two months per year in their home in Maine.

She was diagnosed with relapsing remitting multiple sclerosis (MS) at about age forty. As a result, Jane experienced weakness in her right arm and leg, and was easily fatigued. These symptoms had an impact on her ability to perform at work. (It's also worth mentioning that she had a history of four miscarriages prior to the conception of their one child, and a history of insomnia and constipation.)

Jane wanted to address her energy and weight loss, as the wedding was rapidly approaching. We started her on low dose naltrexone (LDN) and a peptide called dihexa, with which I'd had some success previously in another patient with MS.[12] Unfortunately, Jane did not follow suit, so I decided to take a different tack. I addressed the immune response resulting in breakdown of the superhighway conducting nerve signals from her brain to her limbs.[13] Keeping her on LDN, I added the peptide thymosin alpha-1 (TA-1), an immune modulator, providing restoration of the balance of inflammation and anti-inflammatory response her brain needed. We prescribed rectal butyrate for her chronic constipation, which allowed her to have normal, daily bowel movements. She was able to go back to barre classes without being "wiped out" for days afterward. Her insomnia responded well to oral ketone esters and melatonin. Jane's fatigue improved 70 percent, and she danced the night away at her daughter's wedding.

When We Become Our Own Worst Enemies

Our immune system exists in two forms: the innate immune system, which we're born with, and the acquired immune system. The acquired immunity occurs for most of us around the age of four months, when our bodies realize everything that is ours and stamp it as self; from that point forward, everything we get exposed to gets marked as non-self—an invader.

So, when you come across strep throat at age three, your immune system knows that that's an invader and begins to attack it. For anything unusual or concerning, or any trauma that might occur to your body, the innate immune system is the first responder. The cells of the innate immune system are called macrophages when in the body and microglia when in the brain. These cells have the unique ability to be either Henny-Penny or the janitor; either the sky is falling, everything's terrible, and they're spewing out inflammatory chemicals we call cytokines . . . or they can be quietly putting things away, organizing, cleaning things up, and taking the trash out. They can switch these responses back and forth, based on what's happening in that environment at the time.

Those inflammatory cytokines, like TNF Alpha and IL-6, will tell other macrophages or microglia that something scary is happening, and those macrophages and microglia will begin to create an inflammatory response. In other words, they're sort of the Goosey-Loosey and Turkey-Lurkey of this scenario, aiding and abetting to spread the word.

The immune response should be turned on when there is something scary going on, like an infection or trauma. The problem, however, is when the immune system does not get turned off; then, we see things like peanut allergies, asthma, or mold allergies—those patients' immune systems don't turn off. And that inflammatory response continues, sending out inflammatory cytokines, recruiting the immune system when there is no ongoing danger.

As an aside, if there's an environmental toxin that comes in and damages the cell—like radiation—that damages the cell, those things are going to trigger the innate immune response, too. But for the scope of this chapter, we're focusing on pathogens, bacteria, viruses, parasites, pollen, and the sorts of things that damage the cell itself and can trigger the immune response.

The immune system sees the outside of the cell itself, but it won't see mitochondria, the nucleus, or DNA, because all of those are inside the cell. If there's damage to the cell, its components get released to the space in between the cells. Now the immune system sees it as a foreign invader and begins to create antibodies, much as it would in response to a bacteria or virus. And now you have an immune system response to your own cells. This is one of the ways autoimmune disorders can emerge.

For example, if you're running a marathon and you twist your ankle and tear your deltoid ligament, fragments of damaged cells begin communicating with your immune system, telling it that this is a foreign invader. Your immune system begins to create ligament antibodies, which might be fine, it might not be a problem, and you recover from that without any lingering issues. Or, it might turn into something like rheumatoid arthritis, where your body has an immune response to your own cartilage or synovium, which is the lining of the joint.

This response can also affect your own blood-brain barrier—the barrier between the brain and the rest of your body—if there was damage there. This is the living barrier that protects you from the outside world and protects the brain from the outside world.

What's Happening at the Cellular Level

When we talk about using peptides to restore the useful youthful expression of immunity, what do we mean? Aren't antibodies just antibodies?

Yes, antibodies are antibodies . . . but then there's the thymus gland. T-cells come from the thymus gland, and as we age, the thymus gland gets replaced with fat. This is a process we call *immunosenescence*.

The thymus gland can assist the B-cells to produce antibodies, or it can become the kind of cell that kills viruses and cancer. We call these natural-killer cells. There can be a shift between these two different kinds of T-cells, and it's important for that shift to occur appropriately. For example, when you get a vaccine, you want your body to create antibodies to that vaccine, and once it's done, for the immune system to shut off and rebalance itself so that it can create the virus or cancer-fighting cells as easily as it can create antibodies.

As the thymus gland gets replaced with fat, its proteins that are responsible for communication, like Thymosin Alpha-1 and Thymosin Beta-4, get depleted as well. This causes confusion for the B-cells, which come from the bone marrow. B-cells create antibodies, and they are the last responders—kind of like the FBI that arrive at the crime scene after the fact. If proteins are not there to communicate, B-cells don't know to create antibodies.

There are peptides that can restore or reverse the thymic fat fraction, i.e., how much fat is in the thymus gland itself. If your immune system can be restored to fight off bacteria, viruses, cancer, and aged cells (called *senescent cells*), we may be able to keep you younger, longer.

Let me put it in practical terms. During the pandemic, those most susceptible were the elderly, because their immune systems weren't as strong. The same is true with cancer, COPD, heart disease—older patients are more at risk, because their immune surveillance processes are older and less reliable.

We use peptides, like Thymosin Alpha-1, and Beta-4, to try and restore those immune system signals to tell your body and your immune system to behave in the appropriate way. Our physical body is there to reproduce itself; if it is no longer reproduction-capable, usually past ages thirty-five to forty, then it's going to begin to self-destruct. Why put energy into the immune system if the body is not going to create babies?

Now, your immune system is not good or bad; it all depends on the circumstances it's in. You want your immune system to respond strongly to bacteria and viruses. Attacking these sorts of invaders is an appropriate response, and you want it to shut off as soon as the problem is killed off or removed. If you're exposed to a load of bacteria in your sinuses after having breathed the air of someone who is coughing next to you on an airplane, you want to be able to fight that off quickly, with minimal damage to your body, and then return the immune system to its calm, janitor stage—putting away the antibodies and making the microglia and macrophages calm down.

Very often, symptoms hold the key to whether there may be a problem. Is it a repeated illness or a prolonged, protracted illness? With most viruses, you'll be sick for about three to five days. That's normal. Illness beyond that, particularly prolonged illness beyond that, indicates that there is something going on with your immune system—either something continues to trigger it or your immune system is having difficulty shutting off. Fatigue, for example, is a common symptom of chronic sinusitis or allergies.

Maybe you don't create antibodies in response to a vaccine or an illness. We actually have a test for patients to see what their immune system is doing; we give them a dose of a vaccine and check their blood levels. Some patients don't produce enough, while others overproduce and are in an autoimmune state. In either case, the patient will struggle to fight off illness by not producing the appropriate amount of protectors.

We often think of the immune system as one unit, but it's clearly very complex and there are any number of ways it can go haywire; "Henny Penny" and the "janitor" are two very broad descriptions, along with it being in an antibody-creating state or in a bacterial/ virus fighting state.

This is the reason why you're asked whether you have a fever prior to receiving a vaccine; it's risky to follow through if someone is running a temperature. When your thymus gland has a choice of what to do with its baby T-cells and it commits to a direction, it takes more work and energy to go back the other way. What we need is an immune system in balance, responding appropriately to any circumstance . . . and once that threat is over, it goes back to a balanced state.

So yes, in the face of a virus, you might ramp up your production of virus-fighting cells and ultimately create antibodies, but then afterward, everybody should go back to being calm, normal, and able to respond appropriately again if another invader arrives.

Peptides can be helpful, yes, but they have to be used in the proper sequence and dosing. Peptide therapy isn't always effective in certain cases, like chronic inflammatory response syndrome. In this situation, the immune system is ramped up, typically in response to mold in the environment or specific bacteria (and research is underway to determine whether COVID is also a trigger). About 20 percent of the population has an immune system that just doesn't shut off, continuing to respond (in most cases) to the mold toxins in the environment.

This is different from a mold allergy; this involves the complement system, which I haven't even talked about. Again, it's very complicated. In these patients, the complement response of the immune system does not turn off, so the only way to fix the problem is to remove the person from the environment or remove the mold or bacteria from the environment.

These patients typically have multiple chemical sensitivities. They are sensitive to multiple foods, tend to collect static electricity shocks when they walk across the carpet, and so on. Often, removing them from the environment or removing the problem from the environment so that the exposure is no longer there can work wonders for these patients; however, these patients can also have an adverse response to anything we give them, including peptides.

Peptides can drop their blood pressure or cause them to have a flare of their other symptoms. So we start them on a really low dose, and we take it slowly, trying one thing at a time as opposed to the stacks like we talk about in this book.

Another consideration for these patients is to monitor whether we are inadvertently fueling the problem. If they were to receive a peptide to improve the metabolism of their cells, for example, like the growth hormone secretagogue or a GLP-1, they will receive energy to their immune system, which is going to fuel the problem. So those two, in particular, would not be used, at least in the beginning.

Individual Peptides

These peptides are involved in enhancing and balancing the immune response. They are either naturally occurring or have been slightly modified from the naturally occurring peptide to allow the peptide to evade quick degradation by natural enzymes.

Thymosin Alpha-1

Thymosin Alpha-1 is a natural protein that is produced by the thymus gland, and its production decreases as we age. It's also found to be low in patients who have autoimmune diseases like multiple sclerosis, specifically relapsing, remitting MS.[14] Thymosin Alpha-1 rebalances the thymus gland output, the T-cell, and the binary possibility mentioned earlier (where the T-cell can either trigger the immune system to create antibodies or it can produce cells that are cancer- and virus-fighting). The idea is that the peptide will rebalance the immune system and lower inflammatory cytokines, those chemicals that send out the Henny Penny alerts, professionally known as TNF Alpha IL-6 and others.[15] It can also inhibit the reactive state of those microglia—the immune cells of the brain—so these cells mature into the janitor, therefore reducing excessive activation and instead transition to 'clean up the trash, put things away' mode.[16]

Now, here's another fun fact about Thymus Alpha-1: It can clear viruses, including COVID and hepatitis B, by 86 percent.[17] It also has efficacy in eczema, asthma, rheumatoid arthritis, inflammatory-bowel disease, and Hashimoto thyroiditis, which is an autoimmune disease affecting the thyroid.[18]

I usually prescribe my patients 1.5 mg, administered subcutaneous (SC), taken from daily to twice weekly, depending on the severity of the immune imbalance. It has no known lethal dose and has been studied in children down to 13 months at 40 mcg/kg (micrograms per kilogram).

Melanocortin

There are two of this peptide and both come from the brain: Melanotan-2 and KPV. They bind to melanocortin receptors, which are all over the body. There are several melanocortin receptors, and each one does a different thing. Melanotan-2 is popular among bodybuilders, because it tans your skin. We also use it in patients who are going on vacation, because it also can increase your libido. It tans your skin, it's anti-inflammatory, and it increases libido—what more could you possibly want while on vacation?

Melanocortins reduce inflammatory cytokines, much like Thymosin Alpha-1 does. They reduce the accumulation of an inflammatory cell called a neutrophil. Melanocortin can also decrease excessive production of reactive oxygen species. We'll discuss reactive oxygen species in Chapter Five, but for our purposes here, just understand that reactive oxygen species is a byproduct as you make energy, kind of like car exhaust. A small amount is fine, but too much damages cells. Too little is a problem, too much is a problem, so there is a 'goldilocks' window for where it should be.[19] I will prescribe my patients 200–500 mcg SC twice weekly to daily, titrated to tanning. Occasionally patients will experience transient nausea or diarrhea soon after dosing.

Vasoactive Intestinal Peptide (VIP)

VIP has antioxidant, anti-death, and anti-inflammatory properties. It can up- and down-regulate inflammatory cells as needed and has brain-growth and brain-protective effects.[20] When used to treat Crohn's disease, VIP reduces not only the symptoms of Crohn's but also damage to the intestine that we can only see at the cellular level. So given the histopathology of Crohn's disease, it reduces the inflammatory cytokines like TNF Alpha and IL6.

VIP reduces a food-allergy response and leaky gut, and has been found to regulate the cells that present pathogens and allergens to your immune system.[21] It also protects against the pulmonary effects of COVID.[22]

It can also cause a decrease in blood pressure, flushing, and diarrhea, and you should have your provider check your lipase (a pancreatic enzyme) prior to taking this peptide.

VIP is available either as a nasal spray or injectable. I usually prescribe my patients 50–500 mcg per spray, up to four times daily dosed before noon, as it can cause insomnia if dosed too close to bedtime.

Growth Hormone and Growth-Hormone Secretagogues

The secretagogues are growth-hormone releasing hormones or an analog of growth-hormone releasing hormones, which allow your body to create its own growth hormone so you don't overdose. Why not just take growth hormone directly? Because it can raise your cortisol levels (a stress hormone). And how many of us need that?

Growth hormone mediates development of the thymus gland, so it can improve B-cell response and antibody production. Growth hormone can also improve natural-killer or virus- and cancer-fighting cells, and it can modulate macrophage activity. That means it can restore that T-cell balance and macrophage balance.

It also stimulates production of major antioxidant enzymes so that you don't get an excess of reactive oxygen species.[23] Growth hormone also decreases the secretion of inflammatory cytokines from macrophages.[24]

Peptide Stacks

Presuming a patient does not have chronic inflammatory response syndrome, is dealing solely with an autoimmune process, and we have already addressed their intestinal health, I would add some Thymosin Alpha-1 to their peptide regimen. If they don't mind the tanning side effect, I really like the Melanotan-2, because it binds to melanocortin receptors, decreasing inflammation in general; it is only available by injection, however, while the KPV is available orally.

Most of the time, once a patient receives the first injection, they see that the needle is tiny and can do subsequent injections themselves. Some people just can't get over the needle or the tanning effect, however, so KPV could be used as an alternative.

If a patient has an intestinal inflammatory condition, I like to prescribe them VIP. One spray once a day is a great starting point; then, they can slowly increase their dose up to three sprays daily. (And because our bodies are so intricately woven, they may enjoy better sleep quality, but we'll get to that in Chapter Seven.)

Now if a patient starts with a growth-hormone secretagogue, that's usually a low dose— once a day, five days a week, usually 1.1 mcg/kg of the combination growth hormone-releasing hormone ghrelin agonist: CJC-Ipamorelin. I prescribe it to my patients once a day, with fasting at bedtime five days a week, and then off for two days a week to assist with immunosenescence. Then, I would add Melanocortin and Thymosin Alpha-1.

So if I'm treating Hashimoto's, for example, I would gradually stack Thymosin Alpha-1 and KPV oral. If I'm treating MS, I would stack Thymosin Alpha-1, a growth-hormone secretagogue, and VIP because of how it works on the intestine. For an active viral illness, I would prescribe my patient a much higher dose of Thymosin Alpha-1 and either inhaled or intravenous VIP.

I cannot stress enough that—in any case, but particularly for those with these sorts of immune sensitivities—this is not a one-and-done solution. There will be things encountered in the environment or daily life that will trigger a flare. The flare will have to be treated before returning to regular maintenance routines.

Immune cells can be an ally or they can be a foe. In peptide therapy, making them our ally is always the goal. Your immune system is not, and should not be, your enemy. It is necessary to fight off the daily exposures—yes, daily—to cancers, viruses, and bacteria. These exposures are present in our food and in particles that pass through our respiratory systems and all around us. All of the foreign invaders that come to us every day require a response, and we want our immune systems to respond appropriately and then return to its state of readiness, where it can respond in the best way to get the job done to the next invader.

We want your body to see a cancer cell as a foe and to be able to respond to that cancer with an immune response. Cancer covers itself so the immune system can't see it as a foreign invader, or it suppresses the immune response. This is the reason why elderly patients are more likely to get cancer—their immune systems are suppressed, what we call *immunosenescence*, and they are unable to respond as quickly or efficiently. We want your body to respond to the bacteria or virus that enters your system, but we don't want it to persist when the threat is gone. Peptides improve the youthful expression of your immune response where you appropriately respond to an incoming threat, are able to quickly resolve it, and then quickly restore the natural balance of the immune system.

Final Thoughts

If you are seeking out a functional medicine doctor, ask them how they would treat a bacterial infection. Are they going to give you thirty days of antibiotics? Will they also prescribe you probiotics and other intestinal protection? Are they even aware that there is a concern post-antibiotic therapy? Are they paying attention to the frequency of these infections, looking at why this particular infection has invaded more than once? How would they treat your eczema or allergies—topical steroids? Are they looking for the root cause of your immune system involvement?

Every single cell of our body requires an adequate amount of energy to tackle the jobs that it has to do each day. The immune system, eyeball cells, the heart muscle cells: everything requires a certain amount of energy. When those cells aren't getting the energy they need, you may experience fatigue.

The immune system uses up the largest amount of energy in the body. The T-cells require a tremendous amount of energy to function, so in functional and cellular medicine, a large amount of our focus goes towards that immune system. If we can get the immune system calmed down, often that will fix the fatigue that we face . . . but sometimes that fatigue persists, even though the immune system is rebalanced.

Reactive Oxidative Stress

Oxidative stress is a condition of the cell where it doesn't have enough antioxidants to turn down the reactive oxygen species produced by the mitochondria. As a cell produces energy, it will release this exhaust, which are reactive oxygen species. As we mentioned in the chapter, in small numbers, it's fine... until it gets to be too much.

Your body has a system to take care of that reactive oxidative stress: antioxidants, like Vitamin C, Vitamin E, and glutathione. They are naturally produced by your body. If the amount of reactive oxygen species overwhelms the availability of antioxidants, you get into an oxidative stress state; this is a stress state of the cell that can cause the cell to send out inflammatory cytokine messages to the body.

There's a tattletale inside the cell called nuclear factor Kappa B (NFkB). It sits around the cell looking for scary things, like too much reactive oxygen species, bacteria, and viruses. It will run to the nucleus and say, "Something terrible is happening," and the nucleus begins creating inflammatory cytokines to call the immune system to itself. In response, the immune system says, "Oh my gosh, there's a problem," and it can remain in a state of constant trigger.

Melanocortins can decrease the oxidative stress state of the cell and prevent NFkB from going into the nucleus to trigger the inflammatory response.[25] They are also effective at decreasing the inflammation associated with obesity and diabetes.[26]

KPV is actually a fragment of melanocortins, and it works not only by binding to melanocortin receptors, but also by directly interacting with the DNA itself. This decreases inflammatory cytokines, like TNF Alpha.[27] It also decreases intestinal inflammation and reduces reactive oxygen species.[28]

CHAPTER THREE

Energy

I actually met Melanie at a conference, not as a patient. I was delivering a lecture and she coughed throughout my entire presentation—it was that noticeable from the lectern. Afterward, she approached me, still coughing, and said, "Hey, I need to see you."

"Oh, our practice is currently full," I explained." I'm not taking new patients until next quarter."

"But I'll be dead by then."

Melanie isn't a young person, but she's not ancient—she's in her early seventies, she and her husband run a law practice, and they still work full-time. As we spoke, I noticed that she had no hair on the back of her scalp because she'd had a cancerous spot removed and could barely walk, much less stand, she was so weak. She was also on oxygen. "This started when I got COVID the first time," she explained, and told me that the second time she had it, she was diagnosed with pulmonary fibrosis.

I was starting to believe she was right—she could very well be dead in a few months.

Total Energy Volume and Its Source

Total energy volume is not just how much energy each individual cell has, but the shared amount of energy that the entire component of cells has that they can use for themselves or for each other. For example, when the muscle needs to contract, it takes energy from the liver and the fat cells to actually. Total energy stores are at a whole-body level that can be shared among cells. The brain is one of the highest users of energy; that's why we feel fatigue when our energy level goes down with an infection, an environmental toxin exposure, or poor nutrition or malnutrition. Poor nutrition could be a bigger problem than you may realize. The standard American diet does not contain many nutrients, even though it contains plenty of calories. In fact, I am amazed at the number of times I check blood levels of protein on patients who are morbidly obese, and based on those levels, find they are actually malnourished.

You might be thinking, "I get plenty of protein from burgers, deli meat, and chicken, so I'm good there." In response, I will recount my own experience with nutrition when I was training for a power-lifting competition. I had to watch my macros and was astonished at how things I thought were one macro are actually another.

When we talk about 'watching our macros,' we're talking about a high-level evaluation of nutrients in food, specifically the carbohydrate, protein, and fat content; from there, you change the percentages of those three components relative to one another, based on your training goals or whether you are trying to lose or gain weight.

For example, I always thought that peanut butter was a protein, but it's not; it's actually a fat. I also thought that hummus was a carbohydrate, but it's not—it's also a fat. The goal is to get your macros balanced for your level of activity. A ketogenic diet is 80 percent fat/20 percent protein, or 10/10, or close to that. A carnivore diet is 60 percent fat/30 percent protein/10 percent carbohydrates. There are free online macros tracker apps that can help you figure this out, but a dietitian can also be super helpful.

From there, you can take a deeper dive into nutrients—beyond the high-level evaluation of carb, fat, and protein—that would include more detailed information, like calcium and zinc content. The food that we eat, in general, is really depleted of nutrients unless you're actually growing it in your backyard or you know where it's coming from. It's one of the reasons why I have backyard chickens and a garden with food that is not grown from genetically modified seeds. I know what nutrients are going into the food that I eat, I know what my chickens are being fed, and those are nutrients that I actually want to go in my body. Using a macros tracker, even for a few weeks, can be an easy way to make adjustments in your diet that can make a big impact.

There's just no way to grow huge amounts of crops and get the dense amount of nutrition we need. The ground needs to rest in between seasons, crops need to be cycled, soil needs time to replenish, and that's simply not possible with our nation's food demands. In order to keep up with this demand, cows are fed corn and chickens are fed grains, which is not what they would normally eat. So we are getting a limited amount of nutrients from the nutrient sources that we have, even from our "healthy" food. It's like putting regular gas into the tank of a Ferrari (you are the Ferrari!).

Add to that our country's affection for fats and sugar—soft drinks, fast food, fried food, and so on. That's like putting molasses in that Ferrari tank! Several B vitamins are critical for energy production to occur. If you're eating burgers and fries, and your only vegetable is ketchup, you're probably not getting adequate nutrients to take care of your energy production.

When you start eating farm to table, you will notice a big difference in food flavors, from eggs, to meat, to vegetables and fruits. And when you're over the age of forty, it is critical to get enough protein intake—and it also can be very difficult to do so.

Each cell in your body has a choice of which energy source it's going to use. The cell can use sugar alone, sugar plus oxygen, fat plus oxygen, or protein to make energy. We call energy *nicotinamide adenine dinucleotide* (NAD) or *adenosine triphosphate* (ATP). You must have NAD in order to produce energy; it acts as a precursor but also has other jobs, like DNA repair. Those are packets of energy. Sugar alone makes about two packets of energy, and it's really fast. A cell using this metabolic currency can come up with energy quickly and easily, without much effort on the part of the cell... but it only makes about two packets of energy. We commonly see this happening in a stressed out or cancer cell.

If the cell uses sugar plus oxygen as metabolic currency, it gets about thirty packets of energy for every molecule of glucose. Thirty packets of energy, obviously, is more efficient. It takes a little more work and requires you to put in some energy in order to get that energy out.

Alternatively, fat plus oxygen gives you about a hundred packets of energy. Again, way more efficient, but also a little more time-consuming, because you have to pull the fat from your fat cells and make all these different enzymes to release and burn fat. Sometimes there is fat around the muscles, but usually it's pulled from the liver or the fat cells, and it gets processed by different enzymes than those that process sugar. It can make about a hundred packets of energy, however, so this is way more efficient.

Muscle can be broken down into protein and used as an energy source, but as we age, loss of muscle is expensive in stability, physical performance, and the production of youthful cell signals. As my friend Carl Lanore says, "Muscle is the currency of aging." We don't want to lose the ability of that muscle to produce those youthful packets of energy.

As we exercise, muscle produces myokines, which are chemical messengers that say, "Hey, this is a young body." They announce this to the rest of the cells, signaling them to create proteins from your cells that are also very youthful. This is why exercise is so important—it's telling the rest of the body how to behave.

You need to maintain as much muscle mass as you can as you age, and if you're burning muscle to get energy, it's counterproductive. This is why, when we talk about weight loss, your muscle mass and fat mass should be monitored; it's important that the weight loss is coming from fat, not from muscle.

The energy-generators are called mitochondria, and those mitochondria communicate back and forth with the nucleus—the brain of the cell—telling it what to do and which cells to produce based on how much energy or how much stress the mitochondria are under. The nucleus can say, "Hey, everything's going great. We have plenty of energy." Or it can say, "We're in a stressful state. Please help me by making more mitochondria."

What's Happening at the Cellular Level

Stress at the cellular level depletes energy, either because it's not getting an adequate energy supply to do its job or it has an imbalance of reactive oxygen species to antioxidants. Energy is depleted through:

- infections
- lack of nutrients
- toxins
- cellular overload (of the cell to handle the above)

Many times, we're not aware of infections or toxins in our bodies. We tend to ignore little aches, pains, and sniffles . . . those random sore throats that come and go . . . but then you also feel like you don't have enough energy to get through the day. You feel fatigued or even have brain fog. There are various reasons your total body energy is low; for example, the immune system could be taxed due to a recent infection, and your energy system is trying to recover from having fought this infection. During heavy allergen seasons—spring and fall, when pollen is high—your immune system is revved way up to fight off what it considers a foreign invader, which is pollen.

Even though pollen is not a true enemy per se, your body sees it as a foreign invader and ramps up its immune response . . .and that requires energy.

Many times patients will wonder out loud if they're just lazy and not motivated. They want to sleep all the time and can't get quality sleep. This could actually be attributed to low energy, and we need to figure out what's taking place within the body. We'll address how significant sleep is to recovery in Chapter Seven, but for now, know that without sleep, there is no way for the body to recover.

I usually tell patients to imagine me trying to take care of them in this exam room, but the exam room is full of cardboard boxes. I can still take care of them, but it's much more difficult; I can't hear or see them as well. I have to move boxes in order to get to them to do their exam. It's more energy-consuming to try to do my job with all that trash lying around.

There is an environmental impact on our energy systems, too. Every day, we are exposed to all kinds of things, like parabens and phthalates in our hair, skincare products, metal fillings, and other endocrine disruptors that interfere with the way natural hormones are able to work. They can also interfere with the way the cell is able to make energy, causing fatigue and even difficulty with losing weight.

In my own practice, patients who come to me with these symptoms aren't so much aware or focused on the symptoms themselves; instead, they want to accomplish something and can't figure out why they keep failing. They're the CEO of a large company, or a mother with six children, or a marathon runner, their energy is low, and they can't accomplish whatever it is they want to accomplish.

Women, in particular, need to make the connection between these seemingly random symptoms and their energy levels. As women, we tend to underestimate our value to the world, and sacrifice ourselves to give to others. One of the most important things that others need from us is for us to be happy, find joy, and bring beauty, peace, and creativity to the world. If we are not doing the things that bring ourselves beauty, peace, creativity, and joy, we can't be fully present for others. Let me explain it to you in plain, adaptable terms: Getting a massage, going for a hike, or riding a horse is not selfish if it gives you peace. It is absolutely necessary in order to provide what you bring to the world. We cannot share what we don't have—not authentically, anyway.

Individual Peptides

One of the ways we can reset our metabolic currency to its most efficient state is by using peptides. These particular peptides affect mitochondrial biogenesis—the creation of more energy generators—and some of them are directly from mitochondrial DNA to improve mitochondrial-nuclear communication.

Growth Hormone Secretagogues

Growth hormone secretagogues increase the ability for sugar to enter the cell and be used for energy. There's a receptor on the cell membrane called Glut 4; growth hormone secretagogues increase the presence of Glut 4 on the cell membrane, enabling glucose to enter the cell easily and be used for energy immediately.[29]

The more mitochondria we have, the more energy we can make, and we need to have several enzymes and proteins in place to make this energy. Growth hormone secretagogues increase the proteins needed to make more mitochondria.[30] They increase fat-burning, and remember, fat can produce one hundred packets of energy versus glucose, which produces only thirty. So this peptide can increase fat-burning by 30 percent.[31]

- **Ipamorelin**

For women, we often use ipamorelin—one of the growth hormone secretagogues—alone or in combination with a growth hormone-releasing hormone (GHRH). Usually, I prescribe my patient 1.1 mcg/kg of body weight per day. It must be taken fasting and only five out of seven days per week. I recommend taking the dose at bedtime, if they've given themselves that two-hour window post-meal. If that's really difficult to do, then I would take the dose thirty minutes before dinner or pre-workout. If my patient is concerned about inflammation or weight loss, I will sometimes prescribe it for my patient up to four times per day, as it is very short-acting. Keep in mind, each dose must be taken fasting, so finding that fasting window (two hours after a meal, or thirty minutes before a meal) can be tricky.

- **Tesamorelin**

In lieu of ipamorelin, we might prescribe our patient tesamorelin, which is another growth hormone secretagogue, following the same regimen except for the dosing—500 micrograms for women per day, five days a week. Tesamorelin is long-acting, so it can be used just once a day.

Mitochondrial Peptides

Mitochondrial peptides improve communication between the mitochondria and the nucleus for coordinated action in energy production and cell survival.

- **MOTS-c**

MOTS-c increases fat-burning, increasing the number of packets of energy per molecule, making the cell far more efficient.[32] It also increases NAD and SIRT-1, which improves DNA damage repair and improves the ability of the cell to handle stress.[33]

- **SS-31**

SS-31 also improves SIRT-1 and repairs damaged DNA by lowering inflammatory signals, like tumor necrosis factor alpha and nuclear factor KAPPA B.[34] It improves ATP, NAD, and the overall health of mitochondria; in fact, it can actually restore damaged mitochondria from things like stroke, kidney failure, and a heart attack by way of providing more energy to the cell.

If your cells have the energy they need, they can do whatever they need to do.

Think about what that means at the cellular level, at an organ level, and at a whole-body volume of energy level. If you are feeling tired, it's because somewhere in your body, a cell or an organ is taxed for energy. It's not getting adequate stores.

Peptide Stacks

I put almost all of my energy patients on either a daily regimen of ipamorelin by itself or stacked with a growth hormone-releasing hormone; it just depends on how sick they are. I'll start them on a lower dose if they are particularly ill, or I'll start some of the intestinal or anti-inflammatory things first and then get to treating their energy. Almost all patients benefit from CJC-1295 with ipamorelin, or ipamorelin alone. CJC-1295 is a short-acting GHRH that may be used up to four times a day, but it must be used fasting; its effect is blocked by recent dietary fat or carbohydrates.

Because the mitochondrial peptides tend to be more expensive, I will rotate those whenever possible—one for six weeks, and then flip to the other one for six weeks. I like the cycle of six weeks, because it gives us a bit more time; four weeks isn't quite long enough. We see the benefits that we need to see within six weeks, and people can adjust their systems to it. By that time, we can see how well they will respond. This is a great regimen for patients who have general fatigue.

Final Thoughts

Melanie made tremendous progress in just three months from our conversation at the conference. In addition to receiving peptide therapy, she was walking four miles a day, and her lung function went from 50 percent to 70 percent.

Part of Melanie's success is that she recognized that it's not enough to receive the peptides; as a patient, she had to contribute, too. Using our gasoline analogy, remember regular gasoline will run the Ferrari but not optimally. Energy is probably one of the most critical areas for patient contribution, because if you're not sleeping adequately, getting good nutrients, and doing some form of activity—a stretching exercise, a barre class, or walking around the block—there is no way peptides will improve your energy.

Out of all the body's organs and systems, the brain is one of the highest users of energy. If you don't have adequate whole total body energy, then the brain is going to suffer first. Your ability to think will be impaired, brain fog will persist, you'll have difficulty focusing and finding words if your energy systems aren't working properly and not being addressed.

The Krebs Cycle [include diagram]

The Krebs Cycle is always drawn as a circle, but in the body, it's actually more like a soup. Likely, you forgot about the Krebs Cycle after you took the test on it in high school biology, so a quick refresher: The Krebs Cycle involves several of the enzymes that are inhibited by mercury and/or a lack of nutrients—enzymes that we use to make NAD for the mitochondria. NAD is produced in the cytoplasm in the cell 'soup,' and then it goes to the mitochondria where oxidative phosphorylation is used to produce ATP, the actual energy that's required for things like muscle contraction.

These enzymes typically convert to Acetyl CoA, which is what glucose, fat, or protein become as they get converted to energy. They all have to become Acetyl CoA in order to enter the Krebs Cycle.

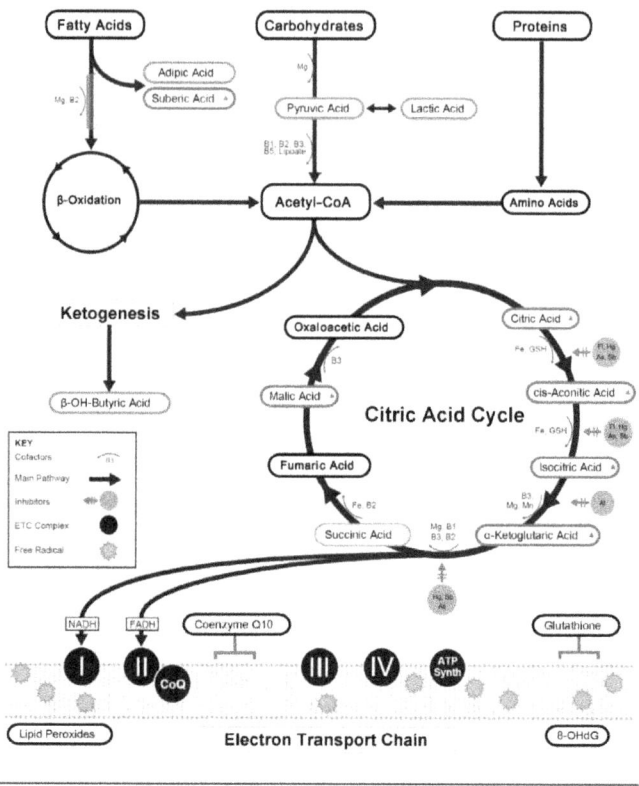

Is Your Doctor Paying Attention?

If you've noticed feeling more tired than your peers and your doctor is not paying attention to it or doing anything directly addressing it, that's a big concern for me. A prescription like Adderall or modafinil—while those have their place—is not the answer to treating fatigue. The solution is figuring out why you're feeling tired and improving the quality of your mitochondria and its function at the cellular level. Questions to consider:

- Is your doctor taking your fatigue seriously?

- Are they doing tests specifically to look at why you are feeling fatigued?
- Are they looking at your sleep?
- Are they looking at your intestinal health, and what you're eating? Are they asking you about your dental health?
- Are they looking at your environmental exposures and personal care products?

CHAPTER FOUR

Cognitive Issues

Elegant, tall, and graceful, Penelope has struggled with elevated blood pressure for years, as had many in her family history. A competitive cyclist and strict vegetarian, Penelope was not interested in using pharmaceuticals to assist with her blood pressure, and as a result, developed some congestive heart failure over time. More recently, she developed some mild cognitive impairment. Given her general overall health, this didn't fit—something was up.

Patients usually don't come to me reporting cognitive impairment, but Penelope was different. She was newly unable to read well, had some difficulty coming up with words, and was concerned about memory loss. In addition to the blood pressure issues, she also inherited a strong family history of ischemic brain disease.

Another patient, Andrew, was also struggling with his mental health. An alcoholic who had been sober for thirty years, Andrew still experienced fairly significant depression and anxiety that he had treated with multiple psychiatric medications, none of which really helped.

In both cases, we needed to rule out other issues. We took steps to optimize their sleep. I looked at their diet and their nutrition status to be sure they were getting adequate nutrients. Using bioidenticals, we optimized and balanced their hormones. These steps were necessary but did little to relieve the cognitive issues with which each patient struggled.

Mental Health Clarification

Depression and anxiety, along with most cognitive impairments, are inflammatory states of the brain. Think about it—none of us has a Prozac deficiency. There isn't a Prozac receptor, per se; it's an inflammatory state. We have to fix cellular function, starting with all the things we have discussed: the immune system, the gut, the ability to make energy. If we can do that, then the cells should begin to function properly.

Once the cells are functioning better, patients can actually optimize their function through peptides. Let me issue a caveat here: that doesn't mean patients can stop taking their antipsychotics or antidepressants. Under no circumstances am I suggesting this happen without the agreement of a licensed psychiatrist or psychologist who knows what they're doing and how it should be done. If their cells are functioning properly and the patient wants to optimize their cellular function through peptide therapy, then they also need to enlist a reputable physician who knows what they are doing. But mental health issues are primarily an inflammatory state and a cellular stress state.

Let me restate: human beings do not have Prozac deficiencies. That's why antidepressants do not work for 30 percent of those who seek treatment for mental health issues[35]—because that's not the problem. And for those who do receive some benefit, the prescriptions often stop working after about a year or so, because it's really just a patch over a much larger issue. That's why dosages are increased, added to, or prescriptions are changed altogether, and the side effects are often intolerable. If we work on fixing the actual problem with the cells—starting with the immune system, the gut, and the ability to make energy—I think we have a way to improve that.

What's Happening at the Cellular Level

Memory loss or cognitive dysfunction is also a form of cellular stress; it manifests from a lack of adequate energy or even an excess of cellular energy. As you make proteins, they require a chaperone that takes them from place to place so that they are doing what they're supposed to do so that it comes out of the nucleus completely formed. This new protein or peptide has to be pruned and folded, sometimes with a different amino acid, fat, or sugar molecule inserted, and sometimes it has to be repaired before it can actually go out into the cell and do its job.

When the cell gets stressed, it creates inflammatory chemicals in response. It recruits the immune system to help handle the stress—to either pack it up and put it away, or cry for help when there's no danger (remember the janitor versus Henny Penny scenario). As trash (those inflammatory chemicals) builds up, cells become even more stressed. Mitochondria are unable to keep up with the demand. The nerves struggle to make connections with other cells; in the brain's case, they can't communicate, memories can't be formed, and things can't be recalled.

Peptides assist with the way that nerve cells work by sending an action potential, like an electrical signal, along the long arm of the cell called an *axon*. That action potential is an electrical gradient that requires a bunch of mitochondria to make all the energy that's required to send that signal along the cell. It also requires the cell to have some construction worker cells called *oligodendrocytes* to maintain a slippery conductive sheath on the outside of the cell. If you don't have those, you develop conditions like multiple sclerosis and others.

Sometimes, that whole process breaks down, and the cell goes through what's called the unfolded protein response—an accumulation of these trash proteins that were improperly folded, or not properly chaperoned, or not properly clipped off, and so on. All that trash buildup of misfolded proteins that we talked about in the previous chapter starts collecting in the cells. The misfolded proteins accumulate and junk up the cell so it's unable to do its job, because a properly folded protein will fit into its specifically designed receptor. If it's improperly folded, it will not fit into the receptor.

Nowhere is this more critical than in the brain, because it can also end up with inflammatory chemicals like excess glutamine. Now if you're already familiar with glutamine, and maybe even take a glutamine supplement, let me reassure you, it's a balancing act: too little or too much is a problem, so what's key is getting the right amount in your body.

Peptides assist with brain function, whether we are awake or asleep. Using peptide therapy, we want to restore the brain cells' ability to take out the trash, grow and divide, make new connections with other neurons, and decrease the inflammatory process that occurs because of trauma or environmental toxins (like alcoholism, traumatic brain injury, infections, or inadequate nutrients—so even specialty diets can be a culprit).

We have seen tremendous results, but I need to underscore that by no means am I suggesting that peptides are a cure for dementia. I have a few dementia patients who have been able to recover some cognition—for example, they could now use a spoon where they hadn't been able to do so before using peptides—but that didn't restore their ability to read and write or resume using a computer. Nonetheless, restoring the ability to use a spoon meant that the patient no longer had to be fed by another person.

Once dementia takes hold, it is really difficult to reverse its impact because the energy systems have already been compromised. The inflammation is already too much. If we can address it at an earlier stage by getting access to the whole body earlier in this process to fix the immune system, fix the energy sources, remove the toxins, improve sleep, and so on, then we can help the cells to prevent things like dementia from occurring. Early peptide intervention can keep things where they are, and maybe even give some reversal.

Peptide therapy needs to work in tandem with a new skill. So before we start on this course of treatment, we ask patients what new skill they intend to learn alongside the peptides to "exercise" their protein-folding (for lack of a better way of putting it). You're not going to build a bicep if you just take a supplement or medication; you have to actually lift the weight to assist whatever you are taking to help you build that muscle. With the brain, you exercise it by learning a new skill.

I can personally attest to the benefits of Dihexa. I have taken it when I had to present two hundred slides, and it helped me recall everything I needed to teach that day. I have taken it in the weeks leading up to a competition to learn a new way of doing something and create new dendritic branching. When I took salsa lessons a couple of years ago, I would take a Dihexa the day of my lesson so that I would be able to retain the steps and create new branching of my brain cells. I was learning a whole new skill that required not only my brain but coordination—the left side of my body doing something different than my right side, and the top half doing something different than the bottom half.

Now there is a difference between occasional forgetfulness and cognitive dysfunction. We've all functioned poorly from lack of sleep, or perhaps we are married to someone with a terrific memory and we tend to count on them to remember things. But if you've noticed a sudden shift and you are unable to recall people's names, form common words, or seem to be in some sort of mental fog, you may be experiencing signs of cognitive dysfunction (not signs of dementia).

I want to underscore again the relationship between our cognitive system and energy and immune systems. If your system is dealing with a lot of inflammation in your intestines, that's going to be communicated to your brain. And those inflammatory cells—macrophages—in the body are going to tell the brain, "Hey, there is an inflammation building up in here." And they will behave in an inflammatory way. In fact, we know that some of the pieces of cell wall of bacteria from the gut are found in the plaques that occur in the brains of patients with dementia. [36]

Inflammation in the gut is not just inflammation in the gut; it's everywhere in the body and affects the entire body. That's why you have to take it seriously. Gut inflammation does not mean that you have dementia, but it also doesn't mean you can ignore it or it could develop into dementia later. Regardless, you do not have to feel resigned to this, or accept something you don't have to accept.

Individual Peptides

Cerebrolysin

Cerebrolysin is a synthetic or bovine-derived peptide combination of brain growth factors and free amino acids. It protects neurons from free radicals, acidosis, and the neurotoxic effects of glutamate, and it improves the metabolic activity of neurons.

Because of its low molecular weight, it can cross the blood-brain barrier if administered subcutaneously (SC), intramuscularly (IM), or intravenously (IV).[37] It can reduce brain toxins like amyloid beta, tau, and the apo E4 variant. It decreases inflammatory cells in the brain. There has been research on its use in Alzheimer's or vascular dementia, mild cognitive impairment, transient ischemic attack, stroke, Parkinson's disease, multiple sclerosis, mood disorders, traumatic brain injury, ADHD, and even in infants as young as six months.[38]

It can be used in combination with TA-1 and TB4 for decreasing the inflammatory response post trauma or stroke, and can also act like calcitonin gene-related protein (CGRP) for pain post-concussion or migraine.[39] Cerebrolysin comes in a glass vial (glass fragments) and can occasionally precipitate (meaning it can start to become solid), so it must be administered through a filter.

Dosing varies depending on the disease being treated from 1 milliliter (mL) SC daily for forty days to 50 mL IV for acute traumatic brain injury (TBI). If given SC, it can cause localized swelling d/t alcohol content and 1 ml volume. For the bovine source, there is theoretical concern about the possibility of transmission of prion disease, which is a brain infection uncommonly found in cows.

Dihexa

Dihexa is a six-amino acid peptide derived from a kidney protein that binds with high affinity to hepatocyte growth factor (HGF), and is multiple orders of magnitude stronger than BDNF but nontoxic and nonneoplastic. It decreases brain inflammation, restores damaged sciatic nerves, and recovers nerves damaged by multiple sclerosis and in clinical trials for ALS.[40] It is antidementia/procognitive, inducing new connections in the brain among nerves HGF.[41]

It is dosed either orally or topically, with the latter applied to the back of the neck at the hairline. The volume of cream required for this is fairly high and often intolerable. Some of my patients will lose weight and need the oral dose decreased from 150 to 50 mg daily or 12–6 mg topically. In my patients, I alternate these every six weeks or so for their nootropic effect and mild cognitive impairment.

Spaden (PE 22-28)

In the face of mood disorders, Spaden (PE 22-28) is a synthetic, long-acting version of the peptide we make that blocks TREK1 channels (a cellular receptor involved in nerve instability and inflammation) and increases the nerve growth factor BDNF. TREK1 channels are responsible for neural stabilization and are associated with depression, atrial fibrillation, seizures, pain, and stroke.[42]

Spaden is available in a nasal spray, and I recommend to my patients two sprays daily for four days, then two sprays twice daily. They sometimes see effects in as short as four days and are able to begin to wean long-acting antidepressants.

L-carnosine

L-carnosine is an over the counter (OTC) oral dipeptide, which serves as a toxin binder and an anti-inflammatory for the brain, with research in autism.[43]

Semax

Semax is a peptide fragment of the hormone ACTH without the hormonal effects of ACTH. Semax binds to receptors in the brain that have been shown to improve learning and memory in animals, increase concentration and attention during information processing, and relieve mental fatigue in humans.[44] Semax demonstrates effects in animals on social stress.[45] Semax has been demonstrated to affect gene transcription to decrease brain inflammation and improve nerve transmission.[46] In this case, it has shown benefit in ADHD, depression, and dementia.[47]

It is available as an injection or nasal spray. I generally prescribe it for my patients on alternating days, along with Selank. Often, I will combine them with L-carnosine oral and alternating cerebrolysin and Dihexa for "brain fog" or post-viral cognitive decline.

Selank

Selank is a peptide fragment of a longer immune modulating peptide. It has strong anxiolytic properties.[48] It affects the way your brain cells transcribe DNA to cause calm.[49]

For my patients with anxiety, this is often a go-to. I usually suggest one spray per nostril intranasal or 300 mcg SC for five to seven days per week via intranasal or injectable administration. Alternatively, I will use it in combination with Semax every other day, depending on the severity of symptoms.

Peptide Stacks

In traumatic brain injury and stroke, we need to add BPC 157. Some athletes take this on a daily basis as a preventive, because most of the research concludes that the maximum benefit occurs if BPC 157 was already in the system before the traumatic injury occurred.[50]

Depression and anxiety are complicated, but they are inflammatory states of the brain. They are just two different expressions of the same disease; the difference is anxiety has a high sympathetic nervous system drive. Thymosin Alpha-1 changes the way the inflammatory process occurs in the brain, so when it's added to this stack, much can be done to ease those issues. Again, I'm not suggesting those who struggle with depression and anxiety stop their prescribed medications, but adding peptide therapy may be a way that a provider could help you treat what's actually wrong instead of the symptoms.

Final Thoughts

Brain health is all about energy, youth, and immune function, factoring in what happens in the intestines and cells' ability to create and use energy. How the cells sense their environment—including the energy status and the inflammatory state of the body—makes all the difference in whether they function properly.

The vagus nerve (located in the cranium and then extends, as the longest autonomic nerve, into the abdominal cavity), in a sense, helps create an electrical and chemical response in milliseconds that results in changes in cellular energy production, changes in organ function, and changes in the microbiome that affect everything from sleep, to sugar-processing by the pancreas, to heart rate, and ultimately, to the development of high-performance . . . or disease. The intestines are intimately connected to the brain by the nervous system, specifically the vagus nerve—the superhighway that gathers information from the intestines, transports it to the brain, and returns the brain's signals back to the intestines—so an inflammatory state of the intestines definitely affects the inflammatory state of the brain. Think about that before you order one more glass of wine, have a fight with your husband, or request a diet soda.

All of those will increase inflammation in the gut and then increase inflammation in the brain.

That second glass of wine may not have a noticeable effect when you are twenty-two, but when you're forty-two, that hangover may affect your entire day. And a hangover is actually toxicity of the brain, i.e., a lack of oxygen; the brain is really stressed out, because it doesn't have the energy it needs, and the immune system is inflamed.

In Andrew's case, he had a history of alcoholism. Even though he had been sober for decades, the repercussions really took effect once he had COVID. We put him on a robust stack of CJC-ipamorelin, Dihexa, and RG-3. Within two weeks, he saw noticeable improvement; all of a sudden, he was interested in playing his guitar again and remembered songs he had written. His creativity increased, and he felt like his depression had vanished.

Penelope started using a combination of peptides that included CJC and a rotation of Dihexa and SS-31, which we prescribed because of her congestive heart failure. Within about six months, she experienced significant improvement, reflected in her echocardiogram and kidney labs, and her cognitive abilities fully recovered.

Regardless of your age and stress level, make sure your doctor is not dismissing your cognitive concerns as "normal aging." They should take your concerns seriously, and actually look into the potential cause and what could possibly be done to reverse it. Are they ordering special tests of blood-brain barrier antibodies? Are they looking into your sleep habits, dental health, and intestinal function to be sure the immune system is properly functioning?

Everyone forgets things at some point, and to some degree, it's true that forgetfulness increases with age. But allopathic doctors don't really have enough tools to get to the root problem; they only have some tools to slow the disease once it manifests.

I hope you are beginning to see that by getting our cells to function properly, and then optimally, we can reverse and eliminate so many chronic issues before they become full-blown disease. There is an efficiency at the cellular level that needs to be addressed, and a lot of things can interfere with that. It sets off alarms that confuse our bodies into thinking we need to fight invaders, accumulate trash, and even gain weight inexplicably.

Peptides give us hope. We have seen many "lost cause" patients recover and restore their health—and their weight.

Yes, Migraine Is a Cognitive Condition

As of this writing, the FDA recently approved several peptides for treating migraines. They're either CGRP -2 antagonists or CGRP-2 inhibitors, or receptor antagonists or inhibitors, meaning they either bind to the natural protein that creates inflammation in the brain or they bind to the receptor so that the inflammatory signal can't get to the receptor.

These peptides have been game-changers for many patients who suffer from chronic migraine. Until this breakthrough, many patients who used prescriptions over a period of time ultimately got worse.

Peptide therapy is an intervention that keeps them from getting worse, because you can put them on a regular regimen. As with most peptides, and unlike most migraine medications, there are no side effects.

Many times, women experience a migraine due to a drop in estrogen, which occurs immediately prior to ovulation at the middle of your cycle and immediately prior to your period. This can be more pronounced in women as they approach menopause. So sometimes, it's a matter of fixing or stabilizing your estrogen.

That's the solution to the problem if you are looking for a root cause, but the other problem can be related to your brain producing an inflammatory chemical called CGRP. There are peptides to help fix that: the daily preventive medicine is called Qulipta, and the abortive therapy is called Ubrelvy or Nurtec. All three have little to no side effects.

CHAPTER FIVE

Weight Loss

Julie was like an octopus; she could juggle many jobs and wear several hats at a time. She had been that way for as long as she could remember.

While she was skillful at engaging others and had an unmatched attention to detail, Julie was also the single mom of an only child, and in the past, she had worked several jobs to make ends meet for them. Finally, she landed a pharmaceutical sales job that not only paid the bills but allowed her to use her skills of party planning and people influencing. Because she was detailed and dependable to her managers and colleagues, she soared to the top of the rankings among her peers.

By age forty-three, Julie began experiencing the gradual onset of brain fog, sluggishness, migraines, constipation, hair loss, chest pain, and a fifty-pound weight gain after a simple viral illness. The following year, she moved to Chicago and took a job as a practice administrator in a large dental office, where she deftly navigated her leadership skills into managing several dentists and hygienists despite her symptoms. She would come home after work and go right to sleep; on the weekends, she'd sleep fifteen full hours and wake up still sleepy. Her weight continued to climb and topped seventy pounds above a healthy weight before she sought our office for help.

We began with an evaluation of her diet, potential food allergies, and environmental toxin exposures. We did an elimination diet, increased her protein intake to maintain her muscle mass, and started her on a regimen of resistance exercise with a trainer three days per week. We balanced her perimenopausal hormones, replaced some missing nutrients, and worked on her sleep and constipation; her excess weight, however, stubbornly remained. By this point, her only child had met the love of her life and the mother of the bride was not going to go to that wedding with an extra seventy pounds!

It's Not Always Calories In, Calories Out

It's no secret that America's waistlines are expanding at rapid-fire pace. The diet and weight-loss industry is expanding, too. So why did I wait until the middle of this book to address something that so many are interested in learning about?

First of all, give yourself a little grace here: weight loss is not all about calories in, calories out—though that is a significant contributor. There are many other factors that contribute to our ability to maintain a healthy weight beyond calories consumed and calories expended. When it comes to weight loss, slow and steady wins the race.

That said, your current 'regular life' needs an honest examination. Are you under chronic stress? What are your food choices? Do you regularly consume alcohol? Are most of your days fairly sedentary? Be honest! Look, my Oura° ring tells me that I sit at my desk for six hours a day, which is a quarter of my entire day. I have to find pockets of time to get up, move around, and use my standing desk if it's going to be one of those particularly busy days. Start moving more deliberately, like getting up every hour to walk around your building or walk up and down a flight of stairs—that is a great starting point to keep your body from getting used to a seated position all day long.

When we gain weight, however, something metabolic is happening, even if it has been triggered by lifestyle choices. We see a lot of patients who regularly consume alcohol, for example. Although we consider it a carb, it is actually a fat—so alcohol will cause inflammation in your body, and therefore, it will cause you to hold on to extra fat. It causes dysbiosis or intestinal bug changes, which will also change the way that your body metabolizes food into pro-inflammatory rather than anti-inflammatory molecules or signaling agents.

Giving up alcohol entirely, or significantly decreasing your intake, will help you lose weight. I realize many of our social settings involve alcohol, but if you are serious about your weight loss, this is one of the big things to give up. Women, especially, associate wine with girls' night out, book club, or just relaxing with friends, and we do ourselves such a disservice this way. There is a lot of evidence associated with alcohol consumption and an increased risk of breast cancer, and I think it is because of the inflammation that happens in the intestines, and then in the whole body, as a result of drinking alcohol.[51]

Weight loss, therefore, should be a long-term strategy. If you have a lot of weight to lose (more than ten pounds), it's really important that you think about this as a one-to-two-year journey that ultimately becomes a lifestyle shift. This is not something that you will be able to do for a little while and then just go back to your 'regular life,' because your regular life is likely the reason why you are where you are.

Peptides can help, but they are not a quick fix. In fact, if you are looking for a quick fix, you may find it—only to be back in the same place you started within a short period of time.

What's Happening at the Cellular Level

When we talk about weight loss, what we are really talking about is encouraging the cell to choose a different substrate for energy; rather than storing energy, we want it to burn that energy. From there, we want it to choose to burn fat as opposed to burning sugar.

If this has been a chronic problem with many unsuccessful attempts at weight loss, it may be some sort of environmental toxin that's standing in the way. We reverse this by getting the immune system on board. You see, when fat cells are under stress, they will begin to enlarge, and as they get bigger, they begin to trigger the immune system.

Having these large fat cells can be inflammatory, which affects the brain and affects the rest of the body's ability to lose fat. This can cause things like diabetes, because—at the cellular level—the cells of the pancreas lose their ability to make energy the way they should. If you are reading between the lines here, insulin resistance isn't solely caused by eating too much sugar; rather, it is the way the cells work and choose their energy source. There are other factors in your life that might interfere with your cells' ability to do that.

For example, if your intestines are a disaster and you are not absorbing nutrients properly, they may send out inflammatory signals all over your body. When that happens, your body is not likely to choose to lose fat, because it's trying to protect you from whatever it sees as a threat.

We have to treat the immune system, and we have to treat the way cells generate and use energy in order to begin talking about weight loss. This concept of how your cells choose to burn fat, how they make a choice in energy sources, and why they might choose another energy source is important to grasp before attempting to re-orient them to make a different choice.

Back in Chapter Three, we talked about how cells make that choice: burning sugar, burning sugar with oxygen, or burning fat with oxygen. When your cells choose the latter, they bring the most bang for their buck—tons of energy for the cell to use at its disposal.

Is there such a thing as too many nutrients? Yes. This is a balancing act—a Goldilocks "just right" environment we are trying to get to—and hyperglycemia (too many nutrients) is a stressor on the body that will also create an inflammatory response.

One of the reasons the body holds onto fat is to protect you from something, whether it's real or perceived: mercury or lead exposure, a persisting infection like Epstein Barr virus, or a mold exposure.

This is why patients can see an increase in their cholesterol. Your body is trying to protect you from that perceived threat or perceived stressor. We have to convince the body to calm down, treat any underlying offender (like an occult dental abscess or low-level dysbiosis), and optimize intestinal function by making sure your microbiome is correct and your motility and absorptive surfaces are ideal. Those things must be balanced in order for you to be in a position to lose weight.

Peptides will help your metabolism function the way it is supposed to in order to optimize body composition and muscle mass for aging. Remember, peptides are signaling molecules; they go to your cells and tell them how to make energy and do the job that they are supposed to do.

Most of the peptides we recommend for weight loss will tell your cells to choose to burn fat as a substrate rather than burning sugar. When you choose to burn sugar, you are not optimizing energy production.

Sometimes, patients have a continuous glucose monitor and can see that their blood sugar is higher in the morning than it was the night before. This is because the liver goes through a process called gluconeogenesis, which creates glucose from whatever it can find, because the cells are, at present, requiring sugar to burn. They will take sugar from your liver, your muscle, or wherever they can to get that energy source that they prefer. We're trying to shift their preference of energy substrate. The cells themselves have to make all kinds of different enzymes to use fat as a substrate, so shifting preference requires a whole rewriting of the script.

Imagine trying a Thai restaurant for the first time and you don't know what to order. Maybe the first time you go, you order something that you don't particularly care for, or it's a really tiny portion and you are still hungry after your meal.

Or maybe you're just not used to the flavors and it's a new experience. Your cells have to adapt similarly to the new signals from the peptides. Their message is, "Hey, it's okay. You need to choose to use fat as a substrate, and start burning it so this person can lose weight."

Does this mean all weight gain is created equal? Setting aside the emotional eating, sedentary lifestyle, messed up immune system, and other environmental factors, *yes*. Looking at weight gain from its most basic, scientific reason, the cell sees that it needs to either protect itself against something or that there is an excess of nutrient intake. Your body will take the easiest route possible, with the least amount of energy input required, to get the most energy output.

In our daily lives, we often do the same thing. We use cars. We shop online. We take elevators. The list goes on. The difference is that, with cells, we can get them to actively change their methods. If you can convert your cells to make the choice to burn fat, then you can burn fat. When this happens, you can usually lose weight, even at rest.

So then there is a bigger question: how do we raise our resting metabolic rate? If you can do that, you can burn fat anywhere from a couple of hours to a couple of days after a workout.

Now, exercise is another topic for another day. There are any number of resources to help you figure out an exercise or workout plan that works for you but understand that it's critical. You cannot expect to lose weight unless exercise is part of your plan, even when using peptides. If you are losing weight and not exercising, you are probably losing muscle mass. And because I firmly believe that muscle is the currency of aging— the way that we help keep ourselves well as we age—then losing muscle mass just to fit into a smaller pant size is not the way to go.

If diet and exercise are not working, however, there may be an underlying cause that is affecting your progress at the cellular level. It's beyond the scope of this book to get into specifics, but you may need to seek out a specialist in mold remediation or a functional medicine specialist in intestinal health who can guide you through restoring that optimal immune function. Or you may need to find someone who can help you with a chronic infection, like Epstein-Barr Virus (EBV) or Lyme disease. Any of those will contribute to a slowed metabolism and the inability to lose weight. If you are pursuing the typical ways to lose weight and they don't seem to be working, you probably need to address those and other environmental factors. Remember, this all starts with your immune system and intestinal health; if your immune system is fighting off what it perceives is a threat, you will not be able to lose weight.

Now here's where it really gets tricky. Weight gain turns right back around and impacts your energy and immune systems. Eventually, fat cells will become their own creators of inflammatory signals. Most of you are familiar with the body mass index (BMI) measurement, a computation based on your height and weight that is loosely correlated with your percentage of body fat. Generally, if your BMI goes over twenty-five, your body begins to create these larger fat cells that are called "white fat." White fat cells have very slow metabolism, and they create a lot of inflammation in the body. Just being overweight can create an inflammatory state!

We also see patients with a high BMI develop insulin resistance, which can progress to diabetes over time. It's all related to these slow-metabolizing, energy-requiring, inflammatory-signaling white fat cells. When we see these patients, they are already in an inflammatory state, especially patients who have a hundred pounds or more to lose. There is a line that's crossed at some point where your body responds by developing these sorts of conditions, and it's purely because of the high BMI. That number is different for everyone; you'll have a high CRP (a general marker of inflammation), and your tumor necrosis factor alpha and other inflammatory markers will be elevated. This is purely because of the production from the white fat cells.

From there, it gets really brutal. The creation of inflammation by the fat cells can then turn around and affect our cognitive functions and create problems with intestinal health. So now we are losing our ability to process, we are losing our good bugs in our gut, and we also can't process nutrients properly, which creates even more inflammation. It becomes a self-fulfilling prophecy that feeds on itself to create inflammation, which creates more inflammation.

Individual Peptides

So, are peptides a cure for weight gain? Do they give us a free pass to just do whatever we want? Okay, I am going to level with you: there is some evidence that suggests they can be what we call exercise mimetics, meaning they can tell your cells that you are exercising even though you're not.[52] To answer the question directly, in some cases, yes. Will you be able to lose a hundred pounds on that? Probably not.

This is going to require effort on your part. Even if the peptides seem to be acting as exercise mimetics, think of how much better they would work if you were actively contributing to your weight loss. It really depends on how much you have to lose, how long you've carried the extra weight, and any other factors that are creating an inflammatory state in your body, causing it to hold on to fat. But the following peptides have been shown to assist in safely losing weight while patients' bodies adjust to the new signaling and messaging about how their cells create and burn energy.

GLP-1

This is an intestinal hormone secreted upon eating. Endogenous GLP-1 induces production of insulin and the proliferation and protection of pancreatic cells.[53] It increases the number of mitochondria (energy generators) per cell and decreases cell death signals in many tissues. GLP-1 protects bone and increases bone density by 16 percent; increases IVF pregnancy rates in obese, polycystic ovary syndrome (PCOS) women; improves cholesterol, blood pressure, CRP, and adiponectin (a fat-burning signal whose absence is consistent with insulin resistance or prediabetes) levels in obese patients; improves kidney function; reduces liver fat without worsening liver fibrosis; reduces heart-related events by 14 percent and all-cause mortality by 12 percent; and reduces pain and inflammation in osteoarthritis.[54]

Endogenous GLP-1 is rapidly degraded by an enzyme called DPP4, which can be inhibited by the ingestion of whey protein.[55] GLP-1 receptor agonists are modified to protect them from degradation—semaglutide is modified to last a week! It works to slow gastric emptying and acid production, so it may cause nausea, reflux, and constipation; it also works at the brain level to increase satiety. GLP-1 improves insulin resistance (i.e., lack of energy in brain cells) and prevents cell death in neurons.[56]

For these reasons, I consider this not only a weight-loss peptide but a longevity peptide. When patients have achieved their goal weight, sometimes they ask about a timeline for stopping their doses. In many patients, I suggest decreasing the dose and continuing, since it has so many other benefits. GLP-1s have been shown to decrease weight by at least 5 percent in over 85 percent of trial participants. Current options are as follows:

- Liraglutide is administered by subcutaneous (SC) injection daily and increased as tolerated (it can cause nausea or constipation) to max 3 mg daily.
- Semaglutide is also administered by SC, but doses are weekly and increased as tolerated to max 2.4 mg weekly. Using a special molecule called SNAC, it can also absorbed orally. Oral semaglutide is dosed while fasting in the morning, at least thirty minutes prior to food intake or other drug consumption, and then you must eat something to initiate its action. Your provider may increase this as tolerated to a maximum of 14 mg.

- Dulaglutide is also SC and taken weekly, and your provider may increase as tolerated to max 4.5 mg.

Tips and tricks for optimizing: follow a low, simple-carb diet, limit alcohol, and stop eating as soon as you feel full. If the nausea is significant, your provider might suggest you decrease the dose by half and dose twice weekly instead of once weekly.

If you are currently also taking a growth hormone secretion (GHS) like CJC-ipamorelin or tesamorelin, your provider may suggest you dose it away from your GLP-1 agonist, as they have opposite effects on growth hormone secretion. In this situation, your provider may recommend a short-acting GHS and GLP-1 agonist and dose them twelve hours apart or on different days, depending on your training schedule.

If the dose does not cause weight loss, your provider may recommend using a GHS five to seven days per week for a month, and then restarting the GLP-1. If weight loss still doesn't occur, your provider should consider food allergies, intestinal dysbiosis, pH balance, cellular oxidative stress, toxic exposures, and nutritional needs.

GIP

This is another naturally occurring intestinal hormone that is released in response to glucose or fat ingestion and works in concert with GLP-1s to raise insulin (in response to a meal and to protect cells of the pancreas). Its effects on fat are still being researched; by itself, it appears to increase fat storage, but in combination with GLP-1s, it causes greater reduction in blood sugar and greater weight loss than GLP-1s alone. It has direct effects on proliferation and protection of the part of the brain involved in memory and bone formation.[57]

Currently, there is one GLP-1 and GIP agonist called tirzepatide available. It is given by SC injection once weekly, and studies show it has greater weight loss with fewer side effects than GLP-1 agonists alone.[58] The pharmaceutical company Amgen has a new product in Phase 3 trials that is a GLP-1 agonist with a GIP receptor antagonist. It appears to be safe, but its efficacy in diabetes and obesity are still uncertain.

AOD 9604

This is a synthetic fragment of human growth hormone involved in lipolysis or fat burning, with no adverse effect on insulin sensitivity as you might expect with intact human growth hormone.[59] Low growth hormone is common in obese humans.

Melanotan II

This is a synthetic fragment of alpha melanocyte stimulating hormone, naturally produced by the brain. Six percent of obesity is due to a genetic variant in aMSH. Melanotan II binds to melanocortin receptors, which are involved in whole body metabolism. In animal studies, it has been shown to decrease appetite transiently and to decrease fat mass in the long run.[60] Potential side effects include high blood pressure, tanning, increased libido, nausea, and diarrhea. Your provider may dose it daily for the first two weeks, and then decrease to twice a week.

MOTS-c

This is a mitochondrial-derived peptide primarily active in skeletal muscle as an exercise mimetic. It inhibits diet-induced obesity, prevents menopausal body weight gain, reduces fat mass, and suppresses inflammatory response.[61] Your provider may prescribe it to be given SC twice per week.

Oxytocin

Oxytocin may be administered intranasally three times per day before meals to assist with eating behavior and metabolism, improve lean muscle mass, and lower LDL cholesterol.[62]

GHRH and Ghrelin Analogues

These stimulate the release of natural growth hormone (GH). GH stimulates fat-burning and release of muscle-building signals. It enhances the uptake of amino acids from the small intestines.[63] It is administered through daily to twice daily SC injections in order to maintain muscle mass in the face of therapeutic caloric restriction.[64]

Tesamorelin decreases visceral fat, and increases lean body mass.[65] Dosing for the short-acting sermorelin, CJC-1295, and/or ipamorelin is weight-based, and usually administered one to three times per day, either when fasting for at least thirty minutes before eating or at least two hours after eating. It is cycled five days on and two days off. Tesamorelin has a longer half-life and only has to be administered once daily. I prescribe this to my female athlete patients on workout days and have them cycle off to a short-acting growth hormone secretagogues. Your provider may dose tesamorelin or CJC-1295 with ipamorelin for synergistic GH release.

Possible side effects of GHS include edema, local skin reaction, allergic reaction, flushing, palpitations, and hypoglycemia.

Peptide Stacks

Let me state that any of these prescriptions would include a higher protein, higher vegetable, reduced calorie diet, and strictly avoiding alcohol at least five nights per week, in tandem with a progressive overload, resistance exercise and HIIT training program.

I use a bioimpedance analysis machine to monitor weight loss rather than a scale, as patients often will lose muscle with calorie restriction, which is not ideal and suggests my patient is not taking enough protein in their diet or adding enough resistance exercise in their lifestyle. Protein intake is easily monitored with one of several macro-calculator apps, which are available on your phone. Fat and muscle mass can be monitored with hydrostatic body fat testing, bioimpedance analysis, or DXA body composition analysis, but both definitely need to be tracked.

A common stack I might prescribe for my weight loss patient would begin with ipamorelin, five days per week at bedtime, increasing to three times daily as tolerated; in women, this may be all you need. After a week or two, I like to add tesamorelin once daily on workout days for a three-month cycle, and then switch to CJC-1295 for a month. Before restarting, I will check their IGF-1 levels to ensure they have not raised too high (>220), and then restart tesamorelin for another three-month cycle. Should they develop an allergic reaction, I would stop and use Alka Seltzer® Gold tabs daily for six weeks, then do a trial of each to see if they tolerate it again.

After another week or two, I would add a GLP-1, like liraglutide daily or semaglutide weekly, depending on the patient's preference and lifestyle. For a woman who works out five days per week, I like using liraglutide as it can be dosed away from tesamorelin/ipamorelin to avoid interfering with their efficacy. If she works out in the morning, I would have her dose tesamorelin/ipamorelin pre-workout, ipamorelin thirty minutes prior to lunch, and liraglutide daily prior to dinner.

If they become nauseated with the liraglutide, semaglutide or tirzepatide may be dosed weekly. We can also try decreasing the dose by half and dose twice weekly to see if the nausea resolves. The ipamorelin can help maintain small intestinal motility while using the GLP-1 to limit nausea and constipation. If the side effects are intolerable, your provider may substitute AOD for the GLP-1 or GLP-1/GIP and dose three times per day before meals with ipamorelin.

For a plateau or for someone unable to exercise, I would add MOTS-c twice weekly for four to six weeks and retest body fat/lean body mass.

Final Thoughts

If you are reading this almost as a last resort, please don't lose hope. You may have tried and tried to lose weight for many years; perhaps you've become resigned, telling yourself that you are just fat and lazy. We know that patients have better success and are more likely to maintain their weight loss if they lose it slowly. The goal is one to two pounds per week or fifty to sixty pounds a year, if you have a lot of weight to lose.

There are also women who have normal bodies with a completely normal BMI, but they're giving themselves a lot of criticism. These women come to me wanting to "lose weight," and it saddens me. I usually tell them, "Your body is perfectly normal. Who's telling you it isn't?"

Comparison is the thief of joy. Our bodies are beautiful, no matter the size or shape, and social media exacerbates our already cloudy judgment about beauty. It's really important that we support one another—maybe even hold one another accountable—to not be so critical of our own bodies.

It's not about being model thin or fitting into a specific size; this is about health. When there is a really high percentage of body fat, your health is in jeopardy. This is where we were with Julie; she was perfectly beautiful, fun, successful . . . and slowly dying. Her health was compromised.

She started by seeing our dietician and working with a trainer who implemented a resistance exercise regimen. We rebalanced her hormones and put her on a little bit of a binder for her toxin exposures. We corrected her thyroid and replaced some nutrients that she was missing. We addressed her intestinal health by prescribing butyrate and tudca, which are synthetic versions of naturally occurring supplements, for her gut.

Then, after getting all that cleaned up, we put her on ipamorelin and prescribed a semaglutide. After about two years, she had lost seventy pounds and kept the weight off; she also looked absolutely radiant in her mother-of-the-bride dress.

Julie is in the gym three days a week for an hour each visit and continues to take daily walks like she did before. Her cognition has improved. Overall, she is able to do and be more than she was able to before. Julie's entire inflammatory state has changed, and by default, it has changed the trajectory of her life.

Again, this is not about the cover of a fashion magazine or being a social media star. This is about health. And since exercising muscle signals to your body that you are not aging, one of the ways we exercise muscle is through resistance training. Once we have achieved a healthy weight, most people want to become leaner and stronger.

They want to optimize.

Insulin Resistance

If you are overweight and your cells are already strained, you are likely what we call insulin resistant, meaning you cannot get enough sugar into your cells to get the energy that the cells need.

When exercising, muscle will actually open up and allow sugar (also called glucose) into the cell without requiring insulin as a carrier molecule. How cool is that? Our bodies have created a way to bypass the absence or resistance of insulin through exercise.

Normally, if you eat a meal and that meal is composed of some protein and some sugar, and your body breaks it all down to amino acids, which will be used for creating proteins and sugar, which will then either be stored or burned for energy. Stored sugar in muscle and liver is called glycogen, and that sugar, once released, requires insulin as a carrier molecule to transport it to your cells. Sugar doesn't go into cells by itself—it has to have insulin to help it through.

When you take in more calories than you are burning, your body will begin to create a condition called insulin resistance. For example, where it may have required one molecule of insulin to get one molecule of sugar across the cell wall, now it requires five molecules of insulin to get one molecule of sugar into the cell across. It becomes less efficient.

When we exercise, the muscle itself can take glucose directly from the bloodstream without requiring insulin. Think about a diabetic who has insulin resistance who requires more and more insulin to handle even a small load of glucose that they eat in their diet. Their blood sugar goes up because they don't have enough insulin to manage the problem. If they exercise, the muscle uses that glucose immediately; it doesn't have to be stored. Even something as simple as going for a walk after a meal can help immediately reduce your sugar levels.

CHAPTER SIX

Human Performance

Melissa came into our practice with hip pain. At fifty-four, she enjoyed traveling all over the world for her job, spending time with her adult stepchildren, and exercising. She was into CrossFit and didn't want to slow down. We sent her to physical therapy, did some injections here in the office, and she still was not back 100 percent, so we ordered her an MRI.

The results revealed that she had a condition called avascular necrosis, where the blood supply withdraws from the end of the thigh bone where it joins the hip bone (or where it meets with the pelvis). With avascular necrosis, the bone begins to die. This condition is common in women around her age, especially those who drink alcohol and are athletic.

Immediately, we got her some nutritional help by adding collagen and butyrate; we took her off alcohol and high-impact activity entirely. She still was walking for cardiovascular exercise, but other than that, she ceased CrossFit with weights. We started her on peptide injections and continued this regimen for about six months. It's fair to say we threw everything at her, because we were trying to save her hip.

What About "Steroids"?

Why would a reasonably athletic person, or someone with age-related aches and pains, consider peptides? In the previous chapter, we talked about increasing muscle mass, decreasing fat mass, and how muscle mass is the currency to keep us from aging; peptides will improve body composition.

If you follow sports of just about any kind, you'll hear a lot about steroids and steroid use. All hormones are steroids, actually, but the ones that are usually headline-grabbers are anabolic steroids—those that cause growth—and there are plenty of those. Testosterone, for example, is an anabolic steroid that can improve body composition. There are testosterone analogs—or what we call selective androgen receptor modulators (SARMS)—that are more or less androgenic, meaning they cause male symptoms like facial hair growth, hair loss on the top of the head, deepening of the voice, and clitoral enlargement in women. A more anabolic SARM would cause growth in general and muscle growth in particular; growth hormone is another anabolic hormone. Testosterone is both anabolic and androgenic, and SARMs can modify the effects, depending on your goals.

When we talk about anabolic hormones socially or read about the latest sports doping scandal in the news, we are really talking about the extra physiologic use of them. If I treat a fifty-year-old patient with bioidentical hormones, I will replace those hormones to the level of when they were forty, for example, not twenty-five. If you are taking them up to that level, that's a supraphysiologic dose—more than what your body would normally make, and maybe even more than what your body would have made at twenty-five. That's where the problem with "steroids" comes in.

I also want to detour slightly here and acknowledge that the World Anti-doping Agency (WADA) does not approve of any peptides whatsoever. So if you are a competing athlete, including Olympians, no peptides are allowed.

When you're talking about medical use versus social use, we are talking about two different things. With peptide therapy, my goal is to assist you with slowing or reversing your aging process—but not to the point I'm creating a monster.

Peptides don't really improve actual strength, per se; their superpower is found in recovery. They improve your post-workout recovery time so you can go to the next workout tomorrow and be able to fully engage in that workout just like you did today versus still needing a little recovery from your workout the day before.

If you are an athlete trying to work out twice a day, you can actually recover from the morning workout and do the second one in the afternoon. That's what peptides allow you to do—train more, which enables you to build more muscle mass, strength, or form to function in your sport.

The Four Types of Athletes

You'll notice that this particular chapter's format is a little different than the others; while the general topic is human performance, there are peptides and stacks that are unique to each of the four types of athletes: endurance, strength, bodybuilding, and mixed. And I will also mention there is a broad range of fitness levels within each type, so I'm not just talking to high-level, competitive athletes—when I say, "athlete," I'm also talking to the guy who swims laps twice a week, the friends who play doubles in a local tennis league, and the woman who just started walking three times a week.

- Endurance athletes are the athletes who are running the entire hour or two of your chosen sport. Think marathon runners, basketball players, and soccer players.

- Strength athletes work on building the strength of the muscle, which is slightly different than the hypertrophy (excessive development) of the muscle in the sport of bodybuilding, fitness, or figure competition. Strength athletes are more like powerlifters, strongmen, and Olympic weightlifters.

- Bodybuilding athletes perform exercises in stacks, meaning they will do three different exercises that all work the bicep, repeat each exercise ten to fifteen times per set, and perform three sets. Each set goes "to failure," meaning that the weight is just heavy enough that by rep number nine or ten, the exercises are very hard or impossible to do. Now, there are several other techniques to achieve muscle hypertrophy or enlargement, but generally speaking, that's how it's done. These athletes are your bodybuilders or fitness/figure competitors.

- Mixed athletes may demonstrate any combination of the above. Decathletes, for example, have to run, throw a shot put, and so on. Gymnasts show quite a bit of strength but must also demonstrate a great deal of muscle control and endurance in the process. Baseball and football players would also be considered mixed athletes.

Regardless of the type or level, however, all four share a common goal: to improve performance.

Peptides and Athletic Performance

So when it comes to peptide therapy and human performance, does one size fit all? No. Different peptides serve different purposes, and there are variations of peptides, timing, and dosing that assist with the specific optimal performance you're seeking.

When it comes to the four types of athletes, there are different needs for each one. Nutritional needs are different. Training needs are different. Each one has a different needs for energy and sustaining it throughout a competition. We also have to consider if we are treating the athlete who is just maintaining or treating the athlete who is competing. All of those require different training and different therapies. It only makes sense that there are different peptides and stacks, based not only on the kind of athlete that someone is but where they might be in their training cycle.

For example, a bodybuilder is going to do what they call a hypertrophy and a cut. They're looking for bulk, so they will be eating tons of the right foods in order to make as much muscle as they can during that time. Then, as they get closer to their competition, they will do a cut, where they decrease their total calories and decrease their percentage of dietary fat in order to lose body fat, making their muscles more defined when they go into competition.

That's why you might meet a bodybuilder who is in a bulk phase who doesn't look like a bodybuilder at all, because they have gained several pounds and lost all the definition in their muscles. They are still training, but their bulk phase delivers all the nutrients possible to their muscles. When they enter the cut phase, they are losing body fat to define those muscles. When you do a bioimpedance analysis on bodybuilders in a bulk phase, they actually have very little visceral fat (fat around their organs). Almost all of their fat is under their skin, what we call subcutaneous fat. When they cut, they change their diet, and you will see them lose all that subcutaneous fat so their muscles look really defined. It's not that those muscles weren't present before; they were just covered with fat.

Strength training goes in cycles, too. There's a high-repetition cycle for a month to six weeks called the repetition phase. You might perform twelve to fifteen reps during this period. Then, you transition to a very small low-repetition phase, known as the strength phase, which might consist of three to five repetitions. They are designed to build on one another so that you're improving your strength as you go. Your peptides follow suit, using a different treatment during the repetition phase than you would use during the strength phase.

So if different peptides give an athlete a certain type of performance edge, how do you approach this with a mixed athlete? It boils down to what they are doing and when—it's still about needs, timing, and dosage. They may change their peptide regimen on a daily basis! It will depend on what they are training on a given day and what cycle of training they are in. And peptides are a part of a whole cadre of modalities—coaches, chiropractor, dietitian, massage therapist, acupuncturist, physical therapist, and so on—to get an athlete to optimal performance.

Peaks and Plateaus

Athletes understand that peptides can assist, but they can't do it all. Peptides can't eat right for them, get enough sleep, endure the training, and so on. All of that still has to happen for athletic performance. And those needs will change, particularly if they hit a peak or plateau.

So much goes into athletic performance—proper recovery, eating right, hydration, quality sleep. When I'm in a training cycle, I have to go to bed by 8:30 p.m. every night. I'm not going out with my girlfriends to have a glass of wine on a random Tuesday night. If you're an athlete paying attention to those factors and you notice that you tire more easily doing the same amount of work, the question is whether this is due to aging or inadequate recovery; and for either answer, the follow-up question is, can we fix that? It's a conversation to have with your provider.

We want to fix the problem, not just treat a symptom or approach this in a roundabout way. A peptide can assist but not necessarily fix, so how do we get to the root cause of why you are feeling stuck? For example, if you feel stuck in a bench press of 115 pounds and you just can't get past it, is this a flexibility problem? Do you need to see a chiropractor? Do you need to do dry needling? Do you need some cupping, a massage, or flexibility training? Is there a stretch class you need to take? Once we address all of those things and you are still having trouble, we might look at some peptides to assist.

Generally speaking, peptides are intended to rejuvenate, improve, or even reverse a particular health issue. Putting that through the lens of athletic performance, is it fair to say that an athlete will not peak, meaning their performance will never decline?

There is a reason why there are age stratifications in competitions. We are most competitive—at our "performance best" as athletes—when we are in our twenties. Past that age, you can still participate in many competitions, but maybe not in the Olympics or at a professional level. Let's say you're in your seventies and still enjoy half-marathons; in certain competitions, you can compete with those in their twenties, but you are less likely to be as competitive with them as you might be with other runners in their seventies. That's why most races have overall winners and age-group winners.

Gender also plays a role, even in endurance sports. Men have physically larger lungs. Even if a man and woman have the exact same height, weight, and body composition, the man will still have larger lungs, and therefore, be able to run longer and faster.

So to answer the original question—yes, there are true plateaus and athletic peaks that occur around the age of thirty. We know that some of it is related to hormone levels and reproductive capacity. Women's bodies are created with the ability to reproduce; during that period, it will have the most immune function, best energy optimization, and best metabolic function. When you were twenty-five, you could eat whatever you wanted, and if you didn't exercise for a month, you could pick it right back up and you weren't even sore the next day. If you tried that at age forty-five, you might be sore for three or four days afterward.

There is also a psychological piece to this. My powerlifting coach always says, "Old weight is easy weight," meaning if I have already lifted 264 pounds, I don't ever have to worry about it again. I have already been there, done that. But 300 pounds? Something would likely get into my head that tells me it's too difficult or dangerous. That something may be a voice of reason or a psychological barrier, and a sports psychologist may be able to help.

What's Happening at the Cellular Level

Your cells want to get the most energy they can. If you're a runner, you want to be able to run for a long time. Your body is going to prepare by providing that substrate (glucose and/or fat) from the liver so that the muscle can continue to contract over and over again. However, in the muscle itself there is only enough energy for about one-two hundredth of a contraction; it has to pull the extra energy from the liver, which has to choose to create that energy from either fat stores or muscle. You want it to choose from fat, if possible—that's the signal we want your own peptides or the peptides that are injected to send.

When you exercise, the muscle pulls sugar from the bloodstream without having to use insulin. In the last chapter, we talked about insulin resistance and the toll it takes on the body. Even taking a walk after a meal can help your body create energy by using the glucose immediately instead of storing it—and bypass some of the need for insulin altogether. Another thing that exercising muscle does that's really cool is produce what we call myokines, those signaling molecules that tell the other cells in the body, "Everything's okay. Nothing to see here," which helps reduce inflammation and unnecessary triggering of the immune system.

An exercising muscle will also improve the number of mitochondria per cell, so we have more energy for brain cells, intestinal health, and, well, overall energy, period. Exercise can help resolve things like fatty liver disease or polycystic ovarian syndrome; improve things like dementia; and maintain things like bone density. Those are secondary reasons why we all need to be exercising regularly, but they're still significant. We don't really think about how critical it is for us to maintain the muscle in our bodies until there is a problem. Simple things like getting up from a chair, reaching for something on a top shelf, or regaining our balance when we stumble will eventually become a challenge if we are not in the habit of regular resistance exercise and stretching. As you age, these little mobility and balance issues could determine whether you'll maintain your independence.

I will often treat my elite athletes very similarly to how I treat my elderly patients: each requires a high amount of protein in their diet, a lot of stretching, and a lot of resistance exercise. They both also need additional services, like massage and chiropractic, to help them maintain. Believe it or not, a lot of the peptides and stacks prescribed for elderly patients are similar to what's prescribed to my elite athlete patients, because their requirements are similar!

Individual Peptides

IGF-1

IGF-1 is produced by the liver in response to growth hormone stimulation. It stimulates muscle growth and protects cardiac muscle, while increasing protein transport into cells and reducing protein breakdown.[66] IGF-1 increases the number of muscle cells and causes glucose uptake by muscle, triggering fat-burning by liver and fat, but it may also cause enlargement of the small intestine and other abdominal organs after prolonged, daily use.[67] Therefore, IGF-1 may be prescribed for my patient in the short-term for five to ten days, two or three days following an injury. It is injected directly into the injured muscle to improve recovery.

MechanoGrowth Factor (MGF)

MechanoGrowth Factor (MGF) is a version of IGF-1 produced locally in response to exercise or damage. It activates stem cells and starts tissue repair/hypertrophy.[68] In rabbits, it is shown to remarkably accelerate ACL regeneration and restore mechanical loading after partial ACL tear.[69] MGF may be prescribed for one to three days immediately following an injury, and your provider may administer it directly into the area of injury.

AOD 9604

We learned about AOD 9604 in Chapter Five. It improves chondrocyte (cartilage cell) production of collagen and is currently in Phase III trials for pain control.[70] In rabbits, when injected intra-articularly, it enhances cartilage regeneration.[71] I prescribe my patients AOD intra-articularly for meniscus/cartilage damage and directly into the injury for tendinitis, ligament strain, and muscle tears.

BPC-157

Previously discussed in Chapter One, BPC-157 heals medial collateral ligament injuries with return of function, organizes collagen, and decreases inflammation.[72] It rescues arthritis; heals muscle tissue after a tear or crush with return to full function; and protects muscle from damage by corticosteroids.[73] This may be prescribed SC in the area of injury and may be administered intramuscular (IM), intratendinous (IT), or intra-articular (IA) directly into the affected joint. Many athletes take it orally every day to prevent significant injury and the effects of traumatic brain injury (TBI). For this, I inject intra-articularly 1.5 mg four times weekly or 200 mcg SC twice daily near the area of injury.

Selank

Selank is a naturally occurring peptide that improves memory, concentration, and emotional tension.[74] It accelerates reaction time, which is helpful for many sports. It also strengthens the immune system, which is critical to an athlete training intensely for competition.[75] This may be prescribed intranasally or SC. I typically prescribe my patients 300 mcg–1 g SC, two to four times per week, for up to three months.

Semax

Semax is a fragment of adrenocorticotropic hormone (ACTH) that raises nerve growth factors and neurotransmitters in the brain.[76] It improves memory and attention and may increase physical performance and adaptation to high-intensity exercise.[77] Semax is one of the peptides that is available SC or IN. I prescribe my patients 300 mcg–1 mg SC, two to four times a week, for up to three months. There are chemists now combining it with SNAC to enhance its oral bioavailability, and that I would dose 500 mcg–2 g.

MOTS-c

In Chapter Five, we learned that MOTS-c is a mitochondrial peptide that improves skeletal muscle as an exercise mimetic.[78] It also improves insulin sensitivity, physical capacity, and motor coordination; increases lean mass regardless of diet; and restores circadian rhythmicity of metabolic flexibility.[79] I prescribe my patients MOTS-c at 4–10 mg SC twice weekly or before competition, as per the stacks below.

Liraglutide

Liraglutide alleviates pain and decreases inflammation in osteoarthritis better than steroids and enhances physical endurance.[80] I dose liraglutide starting at 0.3 mg daily in the morning and increase as tolerated weekly until they reach the goal of 1.2 mg. Liraglutide may cause nausea, which is more likely with alcohol, carbohydrates, or any large meal ingestion. Caution: any GLP-1 may cause weight loss to include muscle mass loss and dehydration, so use of this peptide requires intentional tracking or increase of hydration and protein intake to maintain an optimal state.

Dihexa

Given intramuscularly (IM), dihexa restores sciatic nerve transection.[81] This is available orally or topically, and I usually prescribe my patients 40–60 mg once daily in the morning as it tends to cause weight loss and insomnia if dosed too close to bedtime.

Oxytocin

Oxytocin is a naturally-derived peptide produced in the hypothalamus and released by the pituitary, and is most commonly known for its stimulation of uterine contractions during childbirth. It is also involved in the social bonding of mates and parents. In Chapter Five, we learned its benefits to promote weight loss, but it may also prevent cartilage destruction by decreasing inflammation.[82] It is anabolic to muscle and bone.[83] I prescribe this for my patients to be administered intranasally (IN) 10 U up to four times per day or subcutaneously 40–60 U up to four times per day, but usually after workouts.

Growth Hormone (GH) and Growth Hormone-Releasing Hormone (GHRH)

You're already familiar with GH and GHRH, but maybe not how they are used to optimize human performance.

GH is secreted by a part of the brain called the anterior pituitary in response to exercise and deep sleep; in women, it is released up to nine times per day. Its release is inhibited by a hormone called somatostatin, which is increased by ingestion of fat and carbohydrates. GH stimulates the liver to produce IGF-1, and both somatostatin and IGF-1 are stimulants of somatic growth control. GH affects bone, muscle, carbohydrate, fat, and protein metabolism, sexual maturation, insulin resistance, and immune regulation. For adults with GH deficiency, replacement increases fitness and strength. It also increases sprint performance and VO2max in untrained persons.[84]

In women, use of GH is associated with higher bone mineral density, higher lean mass, and lower body fat as well as fitness in squat jumps and squats.[85] GH increases fat release from intracellular lipid droplets.[86] This release of free fatty acids and glucose initially may appear in blood tests to be insulin resistance but may actually be benevolent hyperglycemia, so your provider may want to monitor your sugar and cholesterol for six months or longer to watch for improvement.[87]

GH may also elevate cortisol or stress hormone, however, and how many of us need that? To counter this effect, we use growth hormone-releasing hormone (GHRH) or ghrelin analogues, which do not raise stress hormone or blood sugar. The combination of the two is more effective than either one alone at raising GH but without the risk of overdose.[88] The first option is sermorelin, which shows improvement in muscle strength and endurance and sleep.[89] It is very short-acting, administered three times daily five to seven days per week by SC injection.

CJC-1295 and Ipamorelin

Next is the combination of CJC-1295 and ipamorelin, usually prescribed together in one solution, which your provider may dose one to three times daily when fasting, five to seven days per week, administered by SC injection. Dosing is weight-based, and I usually prescribe my patients 1.1 mg/kg per dose.

Tesamorelin with Ipamorelin

Somewhat more potent is tesamorelin with ipamorelin. I prescribe tesamorelin for my female patients at 500 mcg and for male patients at 1 mg subcutaneously (SC) once daily five to seven days per week. I will vary this dosing depending on the patient's body size and side effects, like swelling in the hands and localized injection site reaction. I prescribe my patients ipamorelin at 1.1 mg/kg two to three times daily when fasting, five out of seven days per week.

Peptide Stacks

Specific Training Stacks

- For endurance: optimize hormones and diet, then CJC-ipamorelin, BPC-157, TA-1, semax/selank, and larazotide prior to competition.
- For strength: optimize hormones and diet, then IGF-1 after workouts; CJC-ipamorelin cycled with tesamorelin every three months; oxytocin after workouts; and melanotan II for 'off' days.

  When approaching competition, take Dihexa on training days. The day of competition: AOD, MOTS-c.
- For bodybuilding: optimize hormones and diet, melanotan II, and BPC.

  During bulk: IGF-1, CJC-ipamorelin or tesamorelin-ipamorelin, and oxytocin after workouts.

  Approaching competition/cut: maintain protein intake and hydration, then AOD, MOTS-c, semaglutide, melanotan, and larazotide.
- Mixed athlete: optimize hormones and diet, then BPC, CJC-ipamorelin or tesamorelin-ipamorelin, oxytocin after workouts, semax/selank, and melanotan II for 'off' days.

  Approaching competition: maintain protein intake, hydration, and sleep, then Dihexa on training days.

  Day of competition: AOD and MOTS-c.

Other Related Stacks

- Traumatic Brain Injury (TBI): TB4, BPC-157, oxytocin, and SS-31.
- Osteoarthritis: BPC, administered orally or SC, plus AOD 9604 and BPC, or liraglutide intra-articular (IA).

- Tendinitis/muscle tear: IGF-1 twice daily for three days; MGF on days three through ten; then BPC administered both oral and SC or IT; and AOD administered IT.

Final Thoughts

"I'm too old to be active."

"The weight room isn't for me—I don't want to bulk up."

"I have never exercised in my whole life."

I hear these comments and others all the time. My response is always the same: "It's time to start."

The best anti-aging treatment is exercise. If you're over the age of forty, you will benefit particularly from resistance exercise—it is our best ally. This is how we burn fat and maintain muscle, bone, and brain. Stop spending so much time on the treadmill and breaking down muscle with cardio. Remember Sarah from Chapter Five? She lost weight with resistance exercise, because she was operating at that 70 percent of max, which is really where the fat-burning occurs.

Same weight doesn't always equal the same size. Someone who weighs 135 pounds with 40 percent body fat is going to look very different from someone who weighs 135 pounds with 45 percent body fat. They will have a very different shape and fit into a different size of clothing. This is why I'm not a huge fan of the scale itself, because we really need to be looking at body fat and muscle mass and whether someone is in a growth and development phase or death and dying phase.

Do you have fat around your organs? This is called visceral adipose tissue, and is what causes some disease states, like coronary artery disease and fatty liver disease. Excess fat is inflammatory, so you are creating inflammation in the heart, liver, and kidneys, and ultimately, creating diseases like cancer and organ failure. Yet all is not lost.

This can all be improved with resistance exercise, because it will pull fat from everywhere to get you the energy you need for your athletic performance.

Remember Melissa, from the beginning of the chapter? We gave her GHKCU, CJC, ipamorelin, and BPC-157, all as injections. Then we injected her hip with AOD-9604, along with hyaluronic acid and intramuscular pentosan polysulfate.

After six months of treatment, we repeated her MRI. She had complete resolution. They couldn't even tell that avascular necrosis had been present in the first place! Avascular necrosis usually requires a hip replacement; instead, Melissa went back to weight training and is now enjoying powerlifting.

Regardless of our athletic level, however, our muscles and cells need time to rejuvenate. Sleep is a common denominator, because all of us require it for repair and restoration. Our muscles and cells need time to rejuvenate, our brains require sleep in order to do all the things they have to do every day, and our circadian rhythm is intimately tied to how our intestines work and how our brain health is maintained. Without sleep, we lose the ability to do those things well.

Myokines

Myokines are signaling molecules released from exercising muscle that go to other cells in the body and say, "Hey, everything is okay. Calm down, inflammatory immune system. Hey, inflammatory fat cells, calm down. Stop producing so many inflammatory signals." They go to the heart, bone, liver, intestine, and the brain, and they cause things to turn back to, and remain, calm.

This is why we tell patients who are depressed or have diabetes to exercise. We are not just telling you to exercise so that you lose weight; we are telling you to exercise because exercising muscle does so much good.

Irisin is a great example. It encourages the "browning" of white fat so that it is more metabolically active.[90] Plasma irisin levels predict telomere length.[91] Telomeres are the "tails" of the DNA that are gradually shortened with age and are associated with biological aging. Exercise-induced irisin inhibits induction of the inflammatory response in the liver.[92] IV injection of irisin reduces the loss of mitochondria typically caused by insulin resistance or prediabetes and can protect intestinal epithelial cells from cell stress and death due to insulin resistance.[93] It can improve cognition, learning, and memory in brain injury induced by stroke or anxiety.[94] Irisin supplementation induces skeletal muscle growth and hypertrophy.[95] It also regulates bone regeneration and homeostasis.[96] It has been shown to prevent joint cartilage loss and resolve irregular gait when injected into mice eight times weekly.[97] The cool thing about irisin is that it is naturally increased by exercising muscle!

CHAPTER SEVEN

Sleep

Simply put, Elaine personified the phrase "upward trajectory."

In her late thirties, she embarked on a career in accounting. By age forty, she was a CFO, and by fifty, the president of a large industrial company, where she turned their operations around and made it highly profitable. Elaine's career has literally taken her all over the world while carrying the weight of the world—and its many time zones.

Even with all the stress that came from her professional life, Elaine always took care of herself and strived to keep fit. She exercised regularly, did a lot of weight training, and maintained a healthy diet. She and her husband built a lovely life together, complete with a beautiful home, great friends, and healthy family relationships. Although they did not have children, they dote on their dog, Fancy, and Elaine is very close with her nephews, sisters, elderly parents, and stepchildren. She gets together with her girlfriends frequently and gets her hair and nails done weekly—she really seems to have cracked the code of work-life balance.

Still, it's no surprise that at fifty-two, she had not cracked the code on sleep, and it was taking its toll. This had been an eight-year struggle, magnified by perimenopause (the decline in estrogen, progesterone, testosterone, melatonin, and growth hormone starting around age thirty-five) and subsequent menopause. She had tried a lot of different things, including meditation, alcohol, changing her exercise routine, increasing her carbohydrate intake, and over-the-counter sleep aids, like melatonin and valerian root. Eventually, she even tried prescription medications trazodone and Ambien with no real improvement.

These are common avenues many people take. Let me detour here to explain why some of them don't work:

- Alcohol puts you to sleep, but it doesn't keep you asleep. Once the alcohol wears off after about two hours, you wake up wide awake, sometimes with hot flashes, or your sleep is restless. This is actually a common cause of hot flashes in the perimenopausal age group.
- Overtraining can cause insomnia. You are raising your cortisol, and it has a difficult time coming down.
- If you are overtraining and undereating, you will also raise your cortisol and put your cells under stress.
- Many over the counter and prescription medications may yield four to six hours of sleep but not a full night's sleep.

While Elaine was a model of success, she was human, and like most humans, she needed seven-and-a-half to eight-and-a-half hours of uninterrupted sleep each night. The first thing we addressed was her hormones, because that is a common cause of sleep difficulty in women. Once her hormones were balanced, we looked at her diet and exercise regimen, making sure she had adequate nutrition for the degree of workout she was pursuing.

We encouraged her to decrease her alcohol intake to what I call "training mode"—Friday and Saturday only—to give her the optimal time to sleep with the least amount of interference. She decreased her caffeine intake and limited its consumption to take place before 9:00 a.m.

I wanted to be sure she wasn't becoming hypoglycemic in the middle of the night, which would cause her to wake up, so we did a continuous glucose monitor for about two weeks to see where she was. Interestingly, she did have low-blood sugar in the middle of the night that rose high in the morning. This tells me that she was becoming hypoglycemic, probably because she was not consuming enough calories to maintain her degree of brain and exercise activity. When the body senses a hypoglycemic state, it will begin to metabolize or break down muscle to make sugar; by not taking in enough calories, Elaine was defeating her purpose to become stronger, and she was defeating herself by breaking down muscle while she slept. We added half a sweet potato with her dinner and a scoop of resistant starch before bed.

Yes, she had already tried melatonin, but we know melatonin decreases with age. So we had her try it again—not because it helped her sleep but because it helps to reset the circadian rhythm and assists the pineal gland.

Next, we encouraged her to go back to doing some sort of regular meditation practice. Most people abandon meditation because they don't see immediate benefits, don't make it a regular part of their day, and/or "can't seem to get into it." Their minds wander, they think about everything else on their to-do list that day, or they even feel guilty for taking time out to get centered and let their minds 'go blank.' There are a number of apps and tools available that can help, and we gave her a few suggestions to jump-start this practice.

Then we took a careful look at her environment and made some adjustments that would prioritize sleep, starting with her husband seeking treatment for snoring. While snoring is normally associated with sound sleep, it's actually indicative of the opposite—the snorer is not getting quality sleep. Not to mention that, in Elaine's case, her husband's snoring contributed to her lack of quality sleep too. We also set some boundaries for their home life. If her husband was working late, for example, he would not disturb her and instead would sleep in the guest room.

Then, finally, we added some peptides.

Sleep Quality Versus Sleep Quantity

Too often, we joke about making sleep a priority, saying things like, "I'll have plenty of time to sleep when I'm dead!" The problem is lack of sleep can rob you of life in the present—and life in the future.

When I was a surgical resident, part of our training included handling difficult situations responsibly with a lack of sleep. I remember how terrible it was: I fell asleep in a plate of spaghetti while on a date; I would fall asleep mid-sentence, mid-conversation; I would cry all the time. It was debilitating.

Women especially don't prioritize sleep. Whether you have a family of your own or not, we are considered the caregivers of all. We take care of our businesses, our children, other people's children, our husbands, our church family, our friends, our pets—we are the caregivers for everyone, except ourselves. We prioritize ourselves last, underestimating the impact and the value that we have, as women, to the world.

Instead, we focus on everyone else getting better, and fail to realize that what we offer the world is our joy, our creativity, our peace, our patience, our generosity, and our love. Sleep allows us to provide those things to others; if we are not prioritizing it, then we are actually being selfish. We are denying others the opportunity to get the very things they need from us.

In order to be the women that we are intended to be and to be all that we need to be, we have to make sleep a priority. So which is more important: sleep quality or sleep quantity?

After about eight hours, your brain has lost all of its glucose stores and will begin to create ketones. It loves ketones; they really help the brain to function well. Giving yourself that eight hours of sleep can give you a good dose of ketones to help repair and recover from whatever happened the day before.

I have already mentioned that humans require a minimum of seven-and-a-half to eight-and-a-half hours of sleep each night. But if that's all light sleep, you are also not getting what you need. Deep sleep and REM sleep are the rest and regenerate phases that repair and re-organize. When it comes to quality versus quantity, you really cannot separate the two. You need at least four sleep cycles per night to get the full amount of deep and REM that you need.

We'll talk more about these cycles in the next section, but what happens if we don't address the quantity and the quality? Illness certainly begins to occur. We know that cancer is more likely when people don't sleep well, weight loss is almost impossible if you are not sleeping well, and you are also more prone to heart disease.[98]

Sleep is intimately involved in cell repair. If you have an injury, it will be more difficult to recover if you are not sleeping. Without proper sleep, your face will become more wrinkled, because you'll have less collagen and elastin to help maintain healthy skin, and so on.

You've likely picked up on the environment and setting factors through Elaine's story. If you have a partner who snores or keeps a different schedule than yours, you need to agree to set a boundary about this.

Pets and children can also be sleep disruptors. I realize this is a sensitive subject, but if you allow a pet in the room or on the bed while you're sleeping, and they are somehow disruptive, that's affecting your sleep. You need to prioritize this by moving your pet to a different room and telling your child that they are not allowed in your room unless it's an emergency.

What does good sleep look like for most people? In a nutshell, good sleep is seven-and-a-half to eight-and-a-half hours of sleep that is between 25 -to35-percent deep sleep, and 25-to-35percent REM sleep. It's not about quality versus quantity—both are equally important.

What's Happening at the Cellular Level

Your body follows a circadian rhythm; it does certain things during the day, and it does different things at night. In order to conserve energy, your body stops producing enzymes, hormones, and proteins that you don't need at night. For example, it's not going to make digestive enzymes while you are sleeping, because you don't need them— you aren't eating while asleep.

When the brain goes to sleep, it opens up what's called glymphatic drainage pathways. This is like a sewer system for the brain that remains closed during the day. Think about how you create trash during the day—an empty bottle, tissue, take-out food cartons, gum wrapper, milk container, even unwanted food—and what would happen if you had no bin nor means to adequately dispose of all that trash. It would accumulate and rot, attracting pests, some of which carry disease. The brain also creates "trash," and by getting enough good sleep, we allow it time to remove all the trash through the glymphatic system. It drains down into the regular blood system, then the regular lymphatic drainage system, which goes into the inferior vena cava (the large vein that returns blood from the body to the heart). This will leave the body, finally exiting the body in your stool and urine in the morning.

This is why we often want to "sleep on it" when working out a problem or making a decision. While you sleep, the brain is supposed to be organizing and filing all the information that you received during the day. Because you are processing all of that information, your sleep should put you in a fairly heavy state—what we call deep sleep—for the first forty-five minutes or so of sleep. Then you transition into the next phase known as rapid-eye movement (REM) sleep. This is where you have a lot of dreams. You also dream during your deep sleep state, but there won't be a lot of activity; it will be very, very quiet, nothing activity, like looking at an ocean or watching television. REM sleep, on the other hand, is very active; you should be getting 25-to-35-percent REM and deep sleep each, accounting for up to 70 percent of your total sleep every night.

There are different stages of sleep that make up an entire sleep cycle, and you'll run through several cycles throughout the night.

- Deep sleep is the rest and refresh sleep, where you wake up and greet the next day with, *Yay! It's a new day! Where are my pom-poms?*
- REM sleep is where you process all the day's events; you re-file and organize those events, sometimes having dreams about them or about items you didn't process from a time before.
- Lighter-stage sleep lasts about an hour and a half, then you go back into another shorter period of deep sleep, a shorter period of REM sleep, and then back into a lighter sleep.

Again, this cycle happens several times over the course of the night, usually four or five times, depending on how long you sleep. The majority of your deep sleep should occur in the first half of the night.

As you go further into sleep during the night, your heart rate should go down. When your heart rate reaches the nadir (the lowest) point, you should be in the middle of your sleep. Then, it should start to slowly climb as you move towards wakefulness in the morning. If that lowest point occurs later in the night, then you did not have enough time to take out the trash in your brain. We know this by monitoring things like heart rate variability. There are several monitors available you can wear at home.

Other things that can interrupt that middle-of-the-night, lowest heart rate timing:

- Big meal right before bed. Eating your last meal of the day a little earlier is really helpful.
- Alcohol right before bed. You will have a lower heart rate in the beginning of the night, and then your heart rate will go up about two or three hours later. That is counterproductive for the brain to be able to do what it needs to do.

- Blue light before bed. Turn off your screens—laptop, tablet, phone, television, etc. We are designed to go to sleep when it is dark outside and be awake when it's light outside.

Without good sleep, there is no way for the body to recover. Sleep is the time when the glymphatic system opens up and allows the brain cells to get rid of all the trash that has built up during the day—when you have been thinking, working, doing, being, acting, mommy-ing, wife-ing, and bossing. Tons of trash gets built up in the brain cells during the day, and at night, all that trash gets taken out if you get adequate sleep. If you eat or drink alcohol too close to bedtime, your body is too busy digesting all that food and won't spend the energy to clear out the brain, or if you don't get enough sleep, there is inadequate time to clear out the brain. Make sure you cease these activities at least two hours before bedtime, and set aside adequate time for sleep—ideally, between seven and nine hours per night.

If you're not doing that, there is no peptide that is going to help you.

So now that you have a general understanding of why our bodies need sleep, let's get into the details of what is taking place within that quality sleep. There are helper cells in the brain called microglia that can be activated to create inflammation, or they can be calm and act as a janitor, cleaning things up, putting things away in drawers, and organizing the clutter. We want them to be in their calm state; all the things we have discussed so far can help them remain in a calm state. When the glymphatic system opens up, microglia need to be in a calm state, and you get plenty of time and space for sleep.

Because we are supposed to sleep when it's dark and remain awake in the daylight, getting up first thing in the morning and being in the bright sunshine can really be helpful. Not all of us have time to do that, which is where our circadian rhythms get rocked.

I get up at four o'clock in the morning to go to the gym, so it's dark when I leave my house. When I get in my car to go to work, it's dark inside the office. I am in the office until lunchtime, so it might be lunchtime before I actually see sunshine. And that is presuming that it's a sunny day. So admittedly, my own circadian rhythm gets messed up because of my lifestyle. Prioritizing time in front of the sun first thing in the morning is really helpful for a good night's sleep the next night. There are blue lights you can buy and place on your desk during the daytime to give you direct blue-light exposure first thing in the morning.

Another thing that can be challenging, but really helpful, is to maintain calm and focus throughout the day. Whatever activities you need to do, be sure you take a few minutes to relax throughout the day. For me, that may mean taking a moment between patient appointments to sit down at my desk, take a deep breath, pray for them, and release them to God. Then I move on to the next patient. Taking that five minutes between each patient can mean better sleep for me that night. If prayer is not your thing, some other form of meditation or centering may be helpful.

Individual Peptides

DSIP

DSIP is a neuropeptide found in human breast milk and neuroendocrine cells of the pituitary and intestine. It increases delta (slow-wave) sleep. Human studies show that, when given within five hours prior to bed, sleep efficiency and daytime performance are restored to that of normal controls.[99] Do not use it if you are taking a blood-pressure medicine called an ACE inhibitor, like lisinopril or captopril, as this may inactivate the peptide. The active fragment of DSIP is the smaller KND, which has been shown to decrease damage in animal models of heart attack and stroke.[100]

Epithalon

This is a bioregulator (gene-modifying) peptide shown to significantly stimulate melatonin synthesis in older animals in the evening, thereby normalizing the circadian rhythm.[101] I prescribe my patients epithalon for this purpose, dosing at 300 mcg nightly for three or four months.

Oxytocin

Remember this one from previous chapters? It also increases parasympathetic (relaxation) activity during sleep and improves measures of sleep apnea.[102] Oxytocin reduces time to sleep onset, increases sleep efficiency, and increases the percentage of time spent in REM sleep.[103] I prescribe this for my patients to be administered intranasally at 20–40 U before bedtime, up to four times per day for someone for whom rumination is part of their insomnia.

Semax

Here's another one we have looked at in previous chapters. Semax increases resistance to emotional stress, which is helpful in the "winding down" of the day.[104] I also prescribe this for my patients to be administer intranasally, 100–300 mcg per nostril, four to five nights per week.

Selank

This is another bioregulator peptide, which regulates the expression of the GABA(A) receptor—the one to which diazepam, butalbital, and some IV anesthetics bind. I prescribe selank for my patients to be administered intranasally, usually 100–300 mcg, four to five nights per week.

CJC-1295/Tesamorelin/Sermorelin

CJC-1295, tesamorelin, and sermorelin are exogenous GHRH (growth hormone-releasing hormone); they increase non-REM sleep (NREMS). GH stimulates REM sleep.[105] GHRHs promote sleep.[106] I prescribe these for my patients to use at bedtime, fasting at least two hours before injection, with the dosage depending on which you use (all of which have been previously discussed).

VIP

VIP is another peptide we've discussed already. Other benefits to this neuropeptide are that it can restore REM sleep for insomniacs and increases the release of GH.[107] VIP is critical for normal expression of circadian rhythmicity.[108] I prescribe my patients VIP nasal spray for this purpose at 500 mcg in the morning.

Peptide Stacks

For insomnia, I would prescribe my patient DSIP before dinner and a stack consisting of a growth hormone secretagogue (CJC, tesamorelin, or sermorelin) and epithalon before bedtime.

For rumination-induced insomnia, I would prescribe my patient selank, semax, and oxytocin.

For jet lag, semiannual time change, and shift-work sleep disorder, I would prescribe my patient VIP, taken in the morning.

Final Thoughts

Don't forget that as a woman, you have an amazing gift to give to the world. That gift is only available when you are getting adequate sleep and taking care of yourself. Prioritizing and setting boundaries around sleep is not selfish; it's actually selfish to not do that, because we all need you to be at your best self.

Elaine wasn't getting optimal sleep. If she woke up for any reason, she could not go back to sleep. She wanted to fall asleep, stay asleep all night, and wake up in the morning refreshed, and she was struggling to justify "doing all the things" when she wasn't sleeping through the night. Plus, the side effects of things like prescriptions were causing her to feel groggy or dizzy the next morning.

Balancing and optimizing her hormones definitely helped—they gave her a big boost, actually—but all of this still wasn't quite getting her a full night's sleep, particularly when there was a really stressful situation going on. Once we added a few peptides, she was getting a solid seven plus hours of sleep per night. Not only that, her sleep cycles adjusted; almost immediately, she was getting about 25-to-30-percent REM and 25-to-30-percent deep sleep, based on her Oura ring measurements. She is more refreshed, more energetic, and has begun to lose some weight—even though we increased her total caloric intake!

Elaine still has the same personal and professional obligations. But now, she has a firm grasp on all of them because her brain and body can recuperate.

While I hope I have convinced you of sleep's significance to your overall health, some of you may be reading this and think, "Look, losing a few hours' sleep every now and then isn't going to hurt. Everyone has those from time to time." Perhaps if you have a new baby or a late night out, you can recover. But if your sleep is lacking two or more nights a week, this may be a justification for dismissing something that could be chronic. If you have two or more completely sleepless nights per week, consider the fact that sleep deprivation is used as a torture method and reconsider whether you need to see a professional.

Let me underscore sleep's importance. Lack of sleep affects your ability to be creative. It affects your ability to fight off infections. It impairs your executive function, which is thinking through how to make something happen. It affects your decision-making ability. It impairs you to find the right words and general recall of things—people's names, their children's names, and other relationship details. Without proper sleep, you will be more irritable, and it affects your ability to maintain your calm, peace, joy, and gratitude. Next time you catch a cold, consider your sleep patterns and habits.

Your immune system is closely tied to the way that the brain functions; when the brain is full of trash because it didn't get the opportunity to take it out the night before, it will create an inflammatory state. It will signal to the rest of the body, "Hey, things aren't good. Things aren't safe." Your digestion will suffer and conditions like leaky gut may surface. It can also affect your menstrual cycles and fertility, as you will see in the next chapter.

Vasoactive Intestinal Peptide (VIP)

We already know that VIP helps the brain set the circadian rhythm and increases the production of genes involved in the circadian clock. At night, the body shuts off genes involved in digestive enzymes and turns on genes that work on repair. VIP is very helpful to give the body what it needs and when it needs it.

The body needs a lot of energy first thing in the morning to get things going and to do all the things it needs to do—but you have to have energy to make more energy. To set those wheels in motion, VIP increases the production of genes involved in the circadian clock. The body shuts off production of genes that might go towards making digestive enzymes at night, because you don't need digestive enzymes in the middle of the night. So in order to conserve and work efficiently, it uses that energy for something else: repair and restoration.

In the morning, your body turns all those systems back on again, so VIP works to restore that circadian rhythm. It can be very helpful for people who travel across time zones, and if it is given first thing in the morning, it can really jumpstart the body's ability to create the energy it needs at the time you need it to be created.

CHAPTER EIGHT

Infertility, Perimenopause, and Other Female-Specific Issues

Claudine is the sweetest person you could hope to meet. A successful event planner for a professional sports enterprise, she is just genuine, pure joy, all the time, even if she is upset about something, so she has a very diplomatic personality. She has a highly successful career, but also had high hopes for the future—specifically, to be married and have children.

At thirty-two, Claudine had also experienced lifelong painful periods. Her symptoms lasted two, sometimes three, weeks out of every month, starting five to ten days before her cycle and lasting five to ten days after her cycle. After one or two weeks of relief, it would start all over again—abdominal pain, back pain, general body aches, migraine headaches—all related to her menstrual cycle.

Claudine initially sought a polycystic ovarian syndrome (PCOS) specialist for treatment, and he prescribed birth control pills. Later, an ultrasound revealed that Claudine had the classic "string of pearls," which is multiple, small, ovarian cysts. Women are born with a finite number of eggs. Usually, you have one dominant ovarian follicle, where one egg matures every month; that's how you ovulate. They give all the energy, focus, nutrients, and oxygen to that one dominant follicle, then it is released and available to be fertilized. If it's not fertilized, it usually passes with your menstrual cycle.

All those eggs are sitting in tiny cysts all over the ovary, but they are not cystic, like you would see on an ultrasound. Normal egg cysts are just little spaces, little egg houses, in your ovaries. As they fill with fluid and mature—usually, one egg every month in an ideal world—the little egg house enlarges and becomes a cyst. That cyst should rupture, releasing the egg at ovulation, about twelve to fourteen days into your cycle. However, sometimes that cyst does not rupture; it persists beyond ovulation and causes pain and inflammation commonly referred to as an "ovarian cyst."

When you have an ovarian cyst, a syndrome caused by a cyst that does not rupture (i.e., does not ovulate) and persists longer than it should, it creates an inflammatory response that is unrelated to ovulation. The cyst simply persists for no reason; there is no egg to be fertilized. This inflammatory state is why it's painful.

In Claudine's case, she was diagnosed with both endometriosis and PCOS; since she was approaching thirty-five and already had a reduced chance of conception due to her age, these conditions decreased her chances of fertility even more than the average population of women of the same age. Age thirty-five is part of a gradual process; your fertility declines starting around the age of twenty-five, along with other body processes and functions. Your fertility decline lasts until you go through menopause.

Claudine was on several medications for blood sugar, migraines, and pain. Her mother was a patient of mine and asked if I would be willing to speak with her, to see if I could help. Claudine was quite overweight and was struggling to lose the extra pounds. I could offer no guarantees but was certainly willing to talk to her, and two years later, it's been one heck of a journey.

Her first visit was during the pandemic, and I remember talking to her about dating and how interesting it was to date during a time of masking, quarantines, and social distancing. She explained that she might meet someone on one of the online dating sites, where they would have to discuss wearing masks before they ever even met in person. I even remember her talking about meeting the man who is now her husband, and they actually met in person for a coffee. He called her the next day and informed her that he had tested positive for COVID. Thankfully, she did not catch it.

We found out she had Lyme disease, along with a condition called *chronic inflammatory response syndrome* which was triggered by mold exposure in her home and had to move out. Claudine also struggled with insomnia, and she had some intestinal distress, causing her to not absorb nutrients well.

Initially, I performed an assortment of hormone blood work and recommended some detox treatments, along with a book to read about dating and relationships. Of course, Claudine had really high hopes for fertility, but her doctors had told her that, at thirty-two, her chances of getting pregnant were already low. Add to that the fact that she had endometriosis and PCOS (she had endured several painful surgeries to treat her endometriosis, yet it persisted). The odds were not in her favor, but she really wanted to have a baby.

Is It Truly 'Game Over'?

If your doctor is telling you that your symptoms are 'just the way it is' and there is nothing they can do, or if they are telling you to remain on medication until you reach menopause, is it truly game over? Why should we resign ourselves to that? Is it really hopeless?

I have a lot of compassion for allopathic doctors who are seeing twenty-five to thirty patients a day. They don't have the time margin to do the research that I have time to do or that I prioritize doing. Having been that allopathic doctor in the past, I get why this happens. When you're seeing thirty patients a day and each of those patients have ten to fifteen labs that you have to look at, that's hundreds of labs you have to review on top of the patients' appointments, plus all the phone calls that you have to make and/or return. You're lucky to get home by seven o'clock at night, in time to have a bite to eat and go to bed. You might be able to squeeze in some form of exercise on the front or back end of your day but just barely.

I also think the medical training system doesn't encourage curiosity; instead, it encourages you to do what the pharmaceutical companies tell you is possible.

Part of the reason I opened Vine Medical was to persist in finding the absolute best courses of treatment for my patients; if one strategy doesn't work, I'm going to research and find something else. I do not limit myself to what the pharmaceutical companies tell me is available. I research *why* this patient has what she has and see if I can figure out what to do to correct it in order for her to reach her goal.

In Claudine's case, the goal was for her to be able to have a baby. I needed to figure out:

- What was the actual cause of her endometriosis?
- What are the chemicals that interfere with endometriosis resolving, and how could we correct it?
- Was there something else we could do?
- What else could we use to resolve these things, and what else might be triggering?
- Were we able to turn off the triggers so that the whole cascade of inflammation turned off?

What's Happening at the Cellular Level

Right or wrong, the body has a way of correcting itself in certain circumstances—or at least it tries to. When we get sick, it creates antibodies to fight the invader; but as we have already learned, sometimes that goes awry and the body sends itself the wrong signals, creating inflammation and autoimmune disease.

Women struggle with a number of issues that relate back to their hormonal fitness. An imbalance or binding of certain hormones can result in issues ranging from infertility to osteoporosis. The following are some common issues that plague many women and sadly, many carry the pain of these issues privately. But there is hope—more on that later.

Infertility

Now before I dive deeper into infertility, I want to stress it is important that both parties are checked out. Forty percent of infertility or inability to conceive has to do with the male.[109]

As I mentioned, the body tries to correct and protect itself to remain in a state of *homeostasis*, or perfect balance. A female body is not going to allow an unhealthy body to conceive a child, for example, because the goal for the body is to be able to reproduce itself. If the environment is not healthy enough, it will not allow conception. As we age, we become less and less healthy in general; that is one of the reasons everything related to reproduction turns off.

Hashimoto's thyroiditis—where your immune system attacks your thyroid gland—can also contribute to infertility. It is a multifactorial condition that compounds with age.

Another contributor is bacterial overgrowth that can break down your hormones so that instead of clearing the hormones from your system every day, you recycle it. Now your levels are building up instead of being cleared from your intestines.

In a state of inflammation, caused by either infection, environmental stressors, or nutrient deficiencies, the body will spend more of its energy fighting off the problem or repairing or recovering from the problem than it will in creating an environment receptive to reproduction.

Let me put it to you another way: if you are being chased by a bear, you're not going to stop to have sex. And that is essentially what the body thinks is happening when it creates an inflammatory response. It's preparing you to escape the bear, not reproduce.

Now, youth can overcome that—to some degree. That's why younger patients with endometriosis and PCOS, probably younger than we really want someone to get pregnant, are sometimes able to get pregnant. The older you get, the more difficult it will be for you to overcome this problem.

Birth control pills may also be a significant contributor to infertility, which is why some people take them—but when they want to conceive, the pills' lingering effects often stand in the way.

A lot of women are prescribed birth control pills to control symptoms like heavy menstrual periods, painful periods, or even acne. One of the downsides is that birth control pills can shut down the production of your natural hormones. Sometimes it takes months, if not years, to recover from that. Your birth control pills are not natural hormones; they are synthetic hormones that do not resemble the natural hormones that your body makes, meaning they are not bioidentical. They will turn down production of your natural hormones and turn up production of things like sex-hormone binding globulin (SHBG), which binds up other hormones like estrogen, thyroid hormone, and progesterone. Even if your body manages to make those hormones, they will still be bound by SHBG.

This makes *none* of your natural hormones—even if you are making them—available. We don't consider how our organs and systems make use of hormones. Your brain, for example, uses estrogen. The lack of real estrogen and all its effects that the brain needs is one reason why a lot of women who use birth control pills become depressed. That same woman who may be depressed because of her birth control pills shutting off production of estrogen now is prescribed an antidepressant—along with the multitude of side effects it brings with it.

So many things can contribute to infertility. It can be a cellular problem at the ovary level, but sometimes it is a sympathetic nervous system dominance problem. Our autonomic nervous system is composed of the sympathetic and parasympathetic nervous systems. The sympathetic nervous system is the fight-or-flight nervous system, which drives up blood pressure and heart rate when triggered. Ideally, the sympathetic and parasympathetic are in a perfect balance where the body is able to respond appropriately to any situation and then quickly return to a calm, resting state.

The sympathetic system is in constant overdrive for a lot of people, however; in today's world, we all tend to be a bit sympathetic-dominant. There are several things we can do to return to a more balanced autonomic state that are not peptide-related like meditation, gratitude practices, breathwork, contemplative prayer, neural therapy, and using devices like Apollo Neuro and Brain Tap. The nervous system plays a huge role in how the ovaries are willing to respond and significantly contributes to fertility.

Many years ago, there was an interesting study conducted where scientists ordered a pregnancy test on every woman who walked in the door of an OB-GYN practice, following up to see whether they actually became pregnant and carried a child. Approximately 31 percent of pregnancies ended in miscarriage—and the mother never even knew it.[110] When you consider that statistic and the number of times our bodies say, "Nope, not this one; nope, not this one," I think miscarriages happen far more often than we are aware of. When a woman experiences two or more miscarriages, this is recurrent miscarriage, or recurrent pregnancy loss. Both hormone imbalance and genetic variants can result in recurrent miscarriages.

With recurrent miscarriages, the issue isn't getting pregnant, the problem is *staying* pregnant. Improving hormonal fitness can help, and there are also some really simple ways to fix genetic variants.

I also want to state that irregular periods are caused by a number of factors, too. One cause can come from the brain not producing adequate gonadotropin-releasing hormone. Gonadotropins are the hormones released from the pituitary gland, causing the ovary to create estrogen, progesterone, and essentially, the whole fertility cycle.

There may also be a problem at the level of the pituitary, where it's not releasing follicle-stimulating hormone (FSH) and luteinizing hormone (LH). FSH is follicle stimulating hormone, which does just what you would think it would do: stimulates the follicles to mature an egg every month. LH helps to regulate your menstrual cycles. Both should be secreted at specific times during the menstrual cycle, and when they don't, you will have irregular cycles and some fertility problems. These can all be corrected with pharmaceutical variants or natural peptides.

We also see a lot of women athletes who struggle with irregular periods. Once your body fat percentage is low enough, you are not going to create enough hormones to sustain pregnancy; it's part of the body's natural defense. Once it thinks you are no longer of reproductive capability, it's going to begin to turn on the aging process. However, we can give you hormones to help your body sustain pregnancy.

On a happier note, however, we currently have four patients who have gotten pregnant after being told by infertility specialists that there was nothing more they could do when, in fact, we knew there was more that *we* could do—and did.

PCOS

Polycystic ovary syndrome (PCOS) is another condition that can get in the way of conception, which is why it is important for these patients, if they want to have children, to be able to get pregnant as early as they can. Of course, I would never encourage anyone to get married or have children irresponsibly, but it is something to consider if you are an adult with PCOS.

Affected patients will not ovulate often; they will have months and months without ovulation, and their periods will be irregular—a non-ovulatory bleed. This is not a withdrawal bleed, which is when a woman goes through ovulation, doesn't fertilize the egg and, therefore, progesterone withdraws and the lining sheds, also known as menstruation. Patients with PCOS will have an anovulatory bleeding, sort of an overflow of the lining of the uterus. Ultimately, it can become a real problem, because, over time, they can develop uterine-lining cancers. This problem can originate either at the brain level—where they are not cycling their hormones from the brain, which should be giving out estrogen and progesterone in various cycles—or a nutrient or inflammatory problem at the ovary level.

PCOS is also associated with a lot of other hormonal problems with testosterone and cortisol. You can end up with obesity, difficulty losing weight, and blood sugar management problems, like insulin resistance and diabetes. Typically, we will order an ultrasound in those patients to give part of the diagnosis—specifically looking for that string of pearls where multiple eggs are partially matured. We'll also evaluate them with blood tests of all the applicable hormones, nutrients, and inflammatory markers.

Endometriosis

Endometriosis occurs when the lining of the uterus exits the uterus and enters the abdominal cavity. Evidence points to the lining exiting through the fallopian tubes, and those little pieces of the endometrium (the lining of the uterus) will stick to other organs—intestines, bladder, kidneys, or anything else that's in the abdomen.[111] The fragments of secrete proteins that allow them to implant on the ovaries, the uterus, and the outside wall of those other organs.

Endometriosis is a painful condition but is not fatal. It can, however, cause a lot of pain around your menstrual cycles and infertility, among other problems. It is also usually treated with birth control pills, which suppress the natural production of estrogen and progesterone while increasing SHBG to bind up any other estrogen, progesterone, and other hormones that might be present.

Osteopenia, Osteoporosis, and Osteonecrosis

Osteopenia is early bone-density loss, and osteoporosis is significant bone density loss, the latter presenting a huge risk of fracture. These conditions can happen even in young women who have particularly low body fat percentage, but they are more common in women ten years post-menopause.

We usually start screening for these two conditions about age sixty. There are a lot of hormonal factors that may contribute to bone density loss: estrogen, progesterone, testosterone, and thyroid hormone, as well as cortisol. All of these hormones can contribute to bone density, not to mention parathyroid hormone and lack of sufficient Vitamin D. Lifestyle is another contributing factor—the risks are multiplied by a sedentary lifestyle, smoking, and alcohol intake. Young women with anorexia and athletes who overtrain are also at risk.

There is a perfect balance in the body between bone breakdown and bone restoration. This perfect balance allows you to constantly be turning over bone, meaning you are constantly breaking down old bone and replacing it with new bone. Normal, minor trauma to the bone from running, lifting weights, and even walking will help to stimulate this process.

Osteopenia and osteoporosis occur when this process is not in balance. There is either an abundance of bone breakdown or a deficiency in bone restoration, and that all happens in concert with your hormones. Hormonal fitness is a critical piece of treating osteoporosis. The big concern we have about osteopenia and osteoporosis is bone fracture that is not caused by trauma but by daily functioning.

These are typically 'silent' conditions too. Osteoporosis doesn't hurt until you actually have a fracture. If there is no fracture, then the pain is likely not caused by osteoporosis.

The good news is osteoporosis and osteopenia are often reversible. We have many patients who have reversed both by improving their hormonal fitness and diet and participating in a regular exercise regimen—particularly a weight-bearing exercise regimen.

In medical school, we are taught that the only treatments available are pharmaceuticals, and at best, those drugs retain the bone density that remains. Don't get me wrong, there is a place for everything, but do not think that's the place to start.

I think the starting point to treat these conditions is resistance exercise. In tandem, we work on our hormonal fitness and make some dietary changes. Remember, over the age of forty, we need a lot more protein than we think. We live in a world where we are consuming boneless chicken breasts instead of eating chicken off the bone, and so we are missing all that collagen. Our food is cleared of offensive pieces like knuckle bones, and because of these conveniences, we are not getting the collagen that we need.

There is also a lot of evidence that the microbiome is a critical factor in bone density.[112] Because osteopenia and osteoporosis have an association with absorption of nutrients by way of the intestinal microbiome—the healthy bugs being present and the unhealthy bugs not being present—the intestinal epithelial cells need nutrients to be able to properly process the protein that you take in. All of that is critical in the pathogenesis of endometriosis, osteopenia, and osteoporosis.

One of the biggest causes of death with aging is hip fracture, and typically, the age-related osteoporosis will result in a hip fracture of the hip or a compression fracture in the vertebrae.

Elderly patients often do not survive that hit, because they are unable to move around. They change their diet, they change their exercise, their muscles are no longer sending messages to their bodies to be producing, and they age rapidly.

If you are already ninety years of age and have a hip fracture, you don't have a lot of margin for rapid aging. So while the fracture is certainly a risk, the real risk is death.

Sadly, one of the side effects of a lot of the pharmaceuticals that are available to treat osteoporosis and osteopenia is another type of fracture: osteonecrosis, death of your jawbone.

With osteonecrosis, the bone in the jaw begins to disintegrate, a condition that's unique to being on medications for osteoporosis. Think that through: we are treating someone with osteoporosis to prevent them from having a fracture, and one of the possible side effects of that treatment is fracture. Now, many people take these prescriptions and don't experience that problem, but it is common enough—and there are better alternatives.

By propping you and not presenting you with another alternative for treatment, they are creating a situation where you don't have to do the work. They are making assumptions about what you might be willing to do.

Would you be willing to come in every three months and get your hormones checked?

Would you be willing to have someone study how your intestines manage all the nutrients that we take in—including the bugs—and how they process?

Prescriptions for osteoporosis often present a false narrative or, at the very least, do not present the full story. The medication most often prescribed might work for a little while, but it is simply propping up the patient. In a certain sense, these drugs are merely a life-support system that isn't giving you life—they just keep you functioning until something else happens.

Any time I prescribe my patient a pharmaceutical, I will explain to them that it will be used as a temporary measure. These pharmaceuticals will help get them through until we can treat the underlying problem, and then we can wean them off. The what and when depends on how severe the problem is. However, most of the time, I'm not going to use them; I am just going to go ahead and treat the patient's underlying problem.

Remember, the stability of the bone density lies within improvement in bone density, which lies within the stability of bone density—a continuous loop. As much as we want to improve bone density, it's a win if we stabilize bone density, because you lose bone density year after year part of the aging process. If we are stabilizing your bone density, you have actually improved it from where it would have been with a natural aging process.

Treatment of osteoporosis will depend on the patient's willingness to do what is necessary: Are you willing to pick up some weights to do reps and sets consistently? Are you willing to limit your alcohol intake and quit smoking? Are you willing to do some stress management techniques to decrease your cortisol (which is a catabolic or breakdown hormone)?

I read a really cool article where residents who were in an assisted living facility—some of them couldn't even get up out of a chair, some had to walk with a walker or a cane—were enrolled in a progressive resistance exercise program. First, they figured out what their one-rep maximum was. For example, if they were doing a bicep curl and could only curl two pounds, that was the maximum they could lift for one single repetition, i.e. their one-rep max.

For the first week of the program, assuming their one-rep max was two pounds, they went down to one pound, and they worked six or eight sets of six or eight reps, three times a week. The second week, they increased to 80 percent of that one-rep max (in this case, 1.6 pounds). Every two weeks after, they reassessed their one-rep max, and then increased the weight they were lifting by 80 percent. After only eight weeks of training, participants had increased their strength by 174 percent. All the residents who could not get out of chairs initially now could, and those who were walking with assistance were no longer using walkers or canes—and they maintained this level of strength for at least a month after they stopped the exercise program.[113]

Low Libido

Whenever a woman comes to me and says, "My husband doesn't think I have enough libido," one of my first questions is, "Is he taking out the trash?"

Now, a woman's libido is very complicated. It's not just a matter of adequate testosterone; I can give a woman all the testosterone in the world, and it is not necessarily going to turn her on sexually. Women are *diffuse-awareness* creatures, meaning we are aware of everything in the room, everything in the house, and everything in our environment at all times—as opposed to men, who are fairly single-focused. By design, then, women have a difficult time focusing on having sex, but there are things you can do in your relationship to ensure that you are able to achieve *better* focus.

We often describe women's libido as crockpots and men's as gas burners, because you may need your husband to mention to you in the morning, "Hey, I might like to have sex tonight," so that you think about that the rest of the day. We also may suggest you do things that make you feel beautiful, sexy, charming, or engaging . . . whatever those things are to you. Add to that things that help you relax—taking a bath, getting a massage, watching your favorite television show, or whatever allows you to calm down and focus.

And I get it—sometimes that big ol' pile of unfolded laundry that you didn't get to will distract you from being interested in sex. An unmade bed isn't a hospitable environment to entice you into sex. My point is there are a lot of components to low libido that may be unrelated to a hormonal problem. Yes, you need to have hormonal fitness in order to have interest in sex.

And if you are not having orgasms regularly with your partner, you probably will not be interested in sex either—neither would he, if those circumstances were reversed. Making yourself a priority and asking for what you need (both of which are difficult for many women) are also important to libido.

Intimacy is critical for most marriages, and it is critical for satisfying physical intimacy. Intimacy is also important for your body to maintain that youthful age. We know that having sex on a regular basis does a lot of things for your overall health, so making it a priority for you and your partner can be really helpful.

And if all else fails, there's a peptide for that.

If you are experiencing any of these women-specific issues, I want you to be encouraged and excited. This is not the end; you have not received a final decree—there are options. There are things we can do that will restore your hormonal fitness. We can assist in your body doing what it needs to do to allow it to be in a state where a pregnancy is possible, where health and protection of your bones is possible, and where a fulfilling sexual relationship is possible.

Individual Peptides

Kisspeptin

This is a naturally occurring peptide from the hypothalamus and gonads. Genetic variants may lead to hypogonadotropic hypogonadism.[114] Kisspeptin maintains the oocyte (eggs before maturation) pool and regulates oocyte maturation; improves egg implantation and maturation; prevents ectopic pregnancy and ovarian hyperstimulation; increases progesterone; increases natural antioxidants; and finally, its anti-inflammatory effects may relieve endometriosis.[115]

There are several directions I might take with prescribing Kisspeptin, contingent on the strategy and objectives that will benefit the patient. For example, I might prescribe my patient intermittent fasting, resistance training, and/or adding ketone esters or butyrate to trigger my patient's own body's kisspeptin production.

In another instance, I might prescribe my patient low dose estrogen (adminsitered via patch or cream) for stimulation of her own kisspeptin production.

For prevention of ectopic pregnancy or delayed puberty, I would prescribe my patient 1 mcg/kg (100 mcg) per day for six weeks.

For premenopausal secondary hypogonadotropic hypogonadism or PCOS, I would prescribe my patient 1 mcg/kg every day on Day of Cycle (DOC) four through twenty-one for implantation or through DOC twenty-eight if anovulatory (not wanting to ovulate).

There are no known side effects of kisspeptin, except those related to hormones.

Glucagon-Like Peptide-1 (GLP-1)

GLP-1 can increase in vitro fertilization pregnancy rates and decrease free testosterone and ovarian volume in patients with PCOS.[116] It is the peptide your body makes, whereas liraglutide is the synthetic, slightly modified version of GLP-1 that lasts longer. I would prescribe GLP-1 for my patients at 0.6 mg SC daily for two weeks, then increase as tolerated with possible side effects to include nausea, constipation, fatigue, weight loss, and insomnia.

Growth Hormone (GH)

GH acts on the ovary to promote steroidogenesis (production of hormones) and gametogenesis (maturation of eggs), inhibition of follicular apoptosis (death before maturity of the egg), improves the ability of the ovary to respond to luteinizing hormone (LH) stimulation, and activation of thyroid hormone. GH can reinstate normal ovarian activity in GH-insufficient girls and women with delayed puberty or abnormal menstrual cycling and infertility by increasing follicular fluid IGF-1 levels, the number of developing follicles, and the chance of clinical pregnancy.[117] There is no clear evidence of safety of GH-releasing hormones like CJC-1295, tesamorelin, or sermorelin in pregnancy, so duration of use must be with an alternate form of birth control and must be stopped at least two months prior to conception.

Gonadorelin

This is a recombinant human gonadotropin-releasing hormone (GnRH), which stimulates production of LH or follicle-stimulating hormone (FSH). These are hormones from the brain that regulate production of hormones and maturation of eggs. Gonadorelin may be less effective if the patient is overweight; higher doses can inhibit LH/FSH production.

I generally prescribe my patients gonadorelin at 5–20 mcg SC daily on Day of Cycle (DOC) five through ten and again on DOC fifteen to twenty, with the goal of experiencing monthly menses. Patients taking gonadorelin may have side effects of flushing, headache, nausea, or dizziness.

Oxytocin

Oxytocin is a peptide which competitively inhibits gonadotropin-releasing hormone (GnRH) degrading enzymes, so when prescribed mid-menses, it may allow natural GnRH to stay around longer. Oxytocin also prevents ovarian hyperstimulation when used in combination with HCG in fertility treatments, and it inhibits progesterone breakdown to stabilize the uterine lining for implantation of a newly conceived baby. Oxytocin is also an antioxidant, which may help with conditions of inflammation and nutrient stress of the ovary.[118]

I prescribe my patients 5 IU or 10 IU on DOC five through ten for infertility.

BPC-157

Our old friend BPC-157 is a fifteen-amino acid peptide produced in human gastric juice. It has the ability to modulate blood vessel growth signaling with less inflammation, which may help with endometriosis.[119] I prescribe my patients BPC-157 500 mcg twice daily for up to three months.

DSIP

DSIP is an antioxidant and stimulates luteinizing hormone (LH) production.[120] I prescribe my patients 150 mcg SC in the morning for up to three months.

Bremelanotide

Bremelanotide is a small fraction of aMSH (alpha melanocyte stimulating hormone) involved in increasing libido and is FDA-approved for improving female hypoactive sexual arousal.[121] I recommend that my patients take a 2–4 mg injection twice weekly, as tolerated. It can cause nausea in some people and may take up to eight hours for efficacy on the first few doses. Usually by the fifth dose there are no side effects, and the medication is always effective. In some of my patients, dosing on Friday morning is adequate for the entire weekend.

Peptide Stacks

When it comes to the issues we've covered in this chapter, there is no single answer for a single problem. None of these are one-factor problems; they are all multifactorial. All require effort on your part, working in tandem with the benefits of peptides. Peptides are signaling agents that remind cells how to perform, allowing them to do their best job.

For infertility, I would prescribe my patient a stack of CJC-ipamorelin five to seven days a week for three months, then stop for two cycles. After that, we'd follow up with kisspeptin and oxytocin. As these have not been extensively studied in pregnant patients, I recommend my patients pause on fertility attempts for the two or three months of treatment and use a nonhormonal alternate birth control method, like a copper IUD.

For endometriosis, I would prescribe my patient oxytocin, BPC, and DSIP.

For polycystic ovarian syndrome (PCOS), I would start with a stack of CJC-ipamorelin five to seven days a week in tandem with some form of nonhormonal birth control for three months. Then, they would remain off the stack for two months prior to attempting conception.

For patients dealing with osteoporosis and osteopenia, we would start with hormone optimization, collagen supplementation, and resistance exercise. From there, I would prescribe my patient a stack of CJC, tesamorelin, and sermorelin to increase bone density.[122] I would add BPC-157, which aids in healing fractures at levels equal to bone marrow or cortical bone graft; oxytocin, since it is usually low in patients with osteoporosis; and MOTS-c, which improves bone marrow stem-cell function and, ultimately, osteoporosis.[123]

Final Thoughts

"There is hope," I kept telling Claudine throughout the early months of her treatment. Now, she is seeing results—I no longer have to tell her there is hope, because she has it.

We changed out her birth control pills. She was having terrible diarrhea with metformin, which is a common treatment for PCOS, so we switched her to a GLP-1 agonist, a peptide, and we adjusted her hormones using bioidentical hormones. Based on her lab results and her profile, we also addressed her intestinal health and began a simple detoxification protocol.

By fixing her hormones, we fixed her migraines and her pain. Then we discovered that she had some chronic inflammatory response syndrome, probably due to living in a water-damaged building, so as of this writing, we are now in the process of addressing that. Claudine recently married, and she has moved out of her moldy home.

She also lost the excess weight—thirty-eight pounds and counting.

Her goal is still to deliver a baby, and that will be our next step. We have helped many patients who have been told they were 'lost causes,' so there is reason for Claudine to have hope that we can help her there too.

As beautiful as Claudine was, she is now feeling good too, and when you feel good that is on display in your interactions every day.

When you take care of yourself, making you a priority—focusing on sleep, energy, cognitive health, intestinal health, and so on—it will start to show up in your daily interactions and even your physical appearance. When your hormones are aligned, your energy is up, your gut is feeling better, and your insides are percolating, a glow will return that has not been there in a very long time. Yet, you may look in the mirror and think, *Why hasn't my face caught up with the rest of my regained youth?*

Guess what? There are peptides that can assist to create the collagen, elastin, and hyaluronic acid that our body needs to make our skin, hair, and nails look good. Without fillers and without neurotoxins, peptides allow your skin to age yet remain optimally vibrant.

So now that we *feel* better, let's take a closer look at what we can do additionally to make us *look* better.

IUDs and PPIs

IUDs

There are two kinds of intrauterine devices (IUDs). One secretes a little bit of hormone, and the other one does not. The non-hormonal IUD is made from copper, which has a little bit of direct spermicide effect. Years ago, IUDs were a big concern because of the braided string used for extraction that protruded from the uterus. The braided string potentially allowed bacteria to go from the vagina into the uterus, creating a uterine infection. A second concern was the risk of developing toxic shock syndrome, which is a uterine infection related to the IUD being a foreign object. Obviously, these were big problems.

The manufacturer switched the way the strings were made so that they are now a very slick material, and it is much more difficult for bacteria to translocate from the vagina into the uterus. There is still a chance of infection, but it is minimal, and IUDs are more effective than getting your tubes tied at preventing pregnancy.

The downside is if you plan to get pregnant while you have an IUD inserted: you are more likely to have an ectopic pregnancy, meaning the pregnancy implants in the fallopian tubes instead of the uterus. And unfortunately, that pregnancy must be terminated, because otherwise, it will terminate you. As an ectopic pregnancy grows, ot ruptures the fallopian tube, which can cause a lot of illness, including death. But remember, the chances of pregnancy with an IUD are very slim—it is more effective than birth control pills (and to be clear, the only 100 percent sure birth control method is abstinence).

Abstinence aside, the IUD is the best non-hormonal birth control method. The cool thing about the non-hormonal IUD is that your hormones can be adjusted regardless of your birth control method. The hormonal IUD is only good for about five years, but the non-hormonal IUD can last up to ten.

The hormonal IUD should not be used in women who have never had children, as it can cause a scarring problem in the uterus. The hormone that is in the IUD suppresses your body's natural production of progesterone—and this is a real problem. In fact, it's the same problem you have with birth control pills. While it's advantageous because you can regulate your periods and the flow won't be as heavy as before, you are treating it with a non-natural hormone option.

The non-hormonal copper IUD does not have those associated risks. It is a great birth control method for women of all ages, because it is effective for up to ten years. You can use it at age twenty until you are ready to get pregnant; you can use it at age forty until you go through menopause. It is also less expensive than other birth control methods, because you only have to replace it a few times. More importantly, the non-hormonal IUD does not affect the way that your natural hormones perform as other birth control methods can.

With the non-hormonal IUD, we can manipulate your hormones separately. If you have heavy periods, we can give you natural progesterone and work to address other hormonal issues you might be having.

One of the myths that we hear a lot is that IUDs cause a lot of abdominal or period pain. What is common is that women who have been on birth control pills and switch to an IUD have an adjustment to make. The hormonal IUD will function similarly to what they have been used to, but they are still controlling symptoms with synthetic hormones, so the adjustment is minimal. With the non-hormonal copper IUD, women return to whatever their 'normal' period is, but this should not be cause for worry—I manage my patients' terrible periods with other things, like optimizing the patient's hormonal fitness.

PPIs

Proton pump inhibitors (PPIs) are another big cause of osteopenia and osteoporosis. These are found in very common, over-the-counter medicines designed to reduce stomach acid, so check your medicine cabinet; likely, you may have one or two.

PPIs decrease the production of acid in the stomach, but the acid is there for a reason—it helps with digestion. It improves the way our nutrients are processed so that they can be absorbed better. Stomach acid also kills any bacteria that come in via our food.

Those who take PPIs on a regular basis experience recurrent urinary tract infections and, eventually, osteoporosis. Why? They don't have the acid in their stomach to kill off the bacteria as it enters the body, nor the ability to absorb the nutrients from our food to be able to regenerate bone.

CHAPTER NINE

Skin Care and Hair Loss

At fifty-two, Laney was a mom of three, nearly adult, children. She had sold her carpet cleaning businesses and was now an executive coach for owners of carpet cleaning businesses. Laney traveled across the country speaking at industry conferences and had a podcast on business ownership with thousands of followers. She was close to her husband and children; she was also exhausted. She had recently gone through menopause and needed help managing her symptoms.

She was experiencing significant fatigue and could take a nap every afternoon. There was a history of thyroid problems, and she was experiencing hot flashes, among other age-related symptoms—depressed mood, vaginal dryness, and low libido.

Laney was also the type of person who wanted to look her very best. She had Invisalign®, was a lifetime Weight Watchers® participant, and was also practicing intermittent fasting, following the 16:8 method, five days per week. Her weight, however, was creeping up. Remarkably, she slept about seven hours a night and ate clean—all organic, no pesticides or herbicides. She did not have a front-load washer, so there was no mold exposure. And she had no root canal history.

To detour just a bit, front-load washers are notorious for mold. They can spew out their mold spores all around your house. And root canals are a common source of chronic, low-grade infection that may create an inflammatory state in the body.

I did a bunch of blood work on Laney and started her on compounded bioidentical hormones immediately. We talked about making sleep a priority, and her exercise regimen with a focus on increasing her resistance exercise.

Laney's blood work revealed a bit of hypothyroidism and low growth hormone, so we adjusted both. Her blood sugar was a little bit high for fasting, so we put her on a growth hormone secretagogue. Once we put her on that, she felt amazing. She had even lost a little bit of weight. Laney's immediate issues were clearing out, which made her notice a few other things.

"One thing that has always bothered me is that I used to smoke, and now can't put on lipstick without it bleeding into my face," she explained. "And then there are the wrinkles on my face. Is there anything we can do about that?"

The Most Obvious Signs of Aging

We don't always know why we are chronically tired, or why we can't lose weight, or why we have brain fog. But our skin, hair, and nails reflect the most obvious signs of aging. Why?

Most evidence points to the loss of collagen and elastin in the skin, which causes the skin to lose its supple texture, where it used to bounce back to the touch. The loss of the youthful hormones, like estrogen and testosterone, also contribute to wrinkles and hair loss. Our bodies are no longer putting any more effort into making collagen and elastin for beauty, because we are past fertility and, therefore biologically, we are not trying to attract a mate anymore.

There also seems to be a genetic impact where some women develop wrinkles and gray hair earlier than others. And I will also 'state the obvious, about the obvious': there is the environmental component, such as radiation stress from the sun, oxidative stress of the foods we eat, the dehydration from lifestyle choices like smoking and drinking alcohol, pollution exposure, illnesses, and so on.

Infections alone will cause the immune system to spend more energy fighting the infection than making beautiful skin. Immune cells require a lot of energy; if we think about the body as one bucket of energy available to spend every day and you have a virus to fight off, your body will spend that energy fighting that virus rather than creating shiny, colored hair.

Hormone imbalances can cause hair loss as well. Testosterone is a hormone that is present both in men and women, and in the hair follicles on the top of the head, testosterone is converted to dihydrotestosterone (DHT). DHT can cause hair loss on the top of the head for some, including women. It can be prevented by taking a medication that inhibits the enzyme that does that conversion. There are topicals and orals available, but unfortunately, they also tend to affect your testosterone levels, which can result in low libido, low muscle mass, difficulty losing fat, etc.

The skin of the scalp is also sensitive to radiation exposure and environmental toxins, so the top of the head is more likely to become fibrotic. Sunburn, for example, now leaves a scar instead of the skin repairing itself. And a fibrosis is not a place where hair can grow easily.

As your estrogen levels decline, you are more likely to have thinner hair; the follicle itself gets thinner, and that can be multifactorial. Thinning hair can be due to your intestines being unable to absorb the nutrients that you need in order to regenerate hair growth, so even intestinal health affects skin and hair quality.

What's Happening at the Cellular Level

The cells are becoming stressed because they do not have the nutrients nor the energy they need to do their job. As a result, they create this inflammatory state, which either creates fibrosis or crepey skin and sometimes hair loss on the top of the scalp.

All cells, including hair follicles and skin cells, go through a process called *apoptosis*, which is a programmed cellular death. This can be as a result of infection, lack of adequate nutrients, trauma, toxins, etc. Normally, your own stem cells race to the rescue to repair and restore, but if you're noticing your skin getting thinner and you don't heal from wounds as easily, it may be because of stem cell aging and an inability to recover from one of the insults above.

Peptides help at the cellular level, changing the genes to increase production of the more youthful proteins, which increases the energy that is available to the cell enabling it to do what it needs to do. Peptides can revert cells back to their youthful expression versus the survival expression. For example, peptides improve the ability of the intestines to absorb nutrients like protein amino acids from the diet.

So can peptides regrow hair? I have seen it happen. Science has shown they can increase the thickness of the follicle and the number of follicles. It's really fascinating; I have a couple of really great cases of this, and while I did not prescribe my patients peptides alone, they are experiencing wonderful results.

When taking peptides for hair, skin, and nails, are the benefits strictly cosmetic? Or will they help us fight off diseases often associated with aging? One of the peptides under debate is melanotan, a peptide fragment of alpha melanocyte stimulating hormone naturally made by your brain. There is some evidence that melanotan could prevent melanoma, which is an oxidative stress state of the cell. What we have concluded, as a body of researchers, is that melanotan does *not* cause the melanoma, but instead—through tanning of the skin—allows the melanoma to be seen earlier, so that you can see it and get it removed quicker.

Before we move forward and get into specifics, I want to underscore something: you are beautiful just as you are while reading this. I don't care if you are sitting outside under a tree on your lunch break or at home on the couch in your pajamas. If you are reading this, you need to know that you are beautiful, just as you are, this very second, wrinkles, bleeding lipstick, thinning hair, and all.

Individual Peptides

GHK-Cu

This is a bioregulator (less than four amino acids) peptide involved in increasing more youthful expression of genes. It activates wound healing and serves as an antioxidant and anti-inflammatory. GHK-Cu stimulates collagen, activates stem cells for repair, reduces photodamage, tightens loose skin, reduces fine lines and wrinkles, encourages nail growth, fights nail fungus, and grows hair.[124]

I prescribe my patients GHK-Cu in a topical serum at 3 percent with a dermaroller or dermastamp every other week. I also prescribe it systemically in an injectable at 1 mg SC daily for six weeks on and six weeks off. There are no side effects of this peptide, except for the possible effect of copper toxicity, which is visible as a bluish discoloration of the lunule of the nails. Note: GHK-Cu does sting, so often I will prescribe my patients the GHK without copper for hair restoration, as it requires multiple injections into the scalp.

Thymosin Beta 4

Thymosin beta 4 is a naturally occurring peptide of the thymus gland, which influences the growth of blood vessels around hair follicles, activates stem cell migration, and increases speed of hair growth and number of hair shafts.[125]

I administer this into the scalp with other peptides and regenerative therapies at 1 mg, repeated in six weeks as needed.

Melanotan II

This peptide regulates pigmentation of skin for tanning and conditions like vitiligo.[126] I prescribe melanotan for my patients as they approach a beach vacation at 200 mcg SC daily for two weeks. It sometimes can cause nausea, so I often will have my patients start at 25–50 mcg on the first day and increase as tolerated.

Peptide Stacks

As you read through these, I want to remind you that peptides are not a panacea. This is not a facelift; you will not revert to your teenage self. We are, however, talking about aging naturally while improving the way your skin cells appear and the way that they age so that they are healthier, and therefore, we should see a slowing in the rate of visible aging.

For hair restoration, I stack GHK-Cu and Thymosin beta 4 for my patients, with some regenerative therapies injected directly into the scalp. Afterward, I have my patients gently apply the serum to the scalp after a dermaroll or dermastamp twice weekly. From there, I add a growth hormone secretagogue, like CJC-1295, nightly, five out of seven days per week, two hours after a meal, for three months.

For fine lines and wrinkles, I prescribe GHK-Cu to my patients to be applied after a dermastamp on the face, neck, decolletage, dorsum hands, forearms, and distal thighs twice weekly for three months, along with a collagen-vitamin C supplement, like Great Lakes Collagen® taken twice daily.

Final Thoughts

Aging is part of our natural lives. Peptides can assist in the aging process to make things smoother, more graceful, and create an environment that is more conducive to the things you want to do and the things you have to do—but they will not make you a great mother, an amazing CEO, or whatever it is you aspire to be. Peptides are not a magic wand that guarantees those sorts of things; what they can do is help you maintain or regain the youthful expression of your cells. If we are working so hard on the inside of our body to make everything on the inside younger, let's also pay a little attention to the outside. Optimizing *is* a form of self-care.

Hazards of Neurotoxins

I get botulinum toxin, so don't get me wrong, but my take on the problem with neurotoxins is they are neurotoxins—and if they migrate to other parts of the body, you can actually have some permanent neurologic damage that is irreversible.[127] The botulinum toxin can diffuse to several muscles and cause myasthenia gravis-like symptoms, such as double vision, difficulty swallowing, impaired speech, etc.

Another big concern with botulinum toxin migration is memory. The mechanism of action of botulinum toxin affects a chemical called acetylcholine and its breakdown enzyme acetylcholinesterase, both of which are necessary for memory in a part of the brain called the hippocampus.

In a study this year on rats, there was an increase in brain degeneration and presence of inflammatory cells, as well as a decrease in the critical neurotransmitter acetylcholine, in rats treated with botulinum.[128] However, there is conflicting research showing botulinum toxin may be able to reduce release of toxic tau proteins from neurons, so the jury is still out. I encourage you to consider this as you go to your injector for reducing the signs of aging.

CONCLUSION

As we move past our reproductive prime, our body begins to stop production of all the genes that are involved in a more youthful state. We turn off the genes that are involved in reproduction, adequate digestion, muscular fitness, and cognitive performance. All of that happens very gradually, but it starts even as early as age thirty-five. In some women who have conditions like PCOS, it can start as early as their teens.

Peptide therapy provides new opportunities for restoring and turning back on those more youthful genes to resolve age-related issues by using these signals to reignite the more youthful expression of our DNA.

We always start with the gut, because it impacts most of the immune system and a lot of the neurotransmitters. Across the intestinal membrane, which runs basically from our nose down to our anus, is where the majority of our interface with the world occurs. Your immune system being closely linked with your gut health means that it's turned on or off, triggered or not, in response to infection, trauma, or stress, which can cause autoimmune and inflammatory problems right at that interface between the world and your body.

We want to make friends with our immune system, because it can either attack the threats we want it to—or it can attack us. We want to strike a balance in the cells can that either create antibodies or the natural killer cells that fight off viruses and cancers. A dominance on the antibody side results in autoimmune disease, and dominance on the natural killer side makes it so that you're unable to remember the bacteria and viruses in your body, which creates a constant inflammatory state. Everything needs to be in balance to equalize and optimize our health.

Then vs. Now

When we're younger, we are able to get away with a lot more carelessness with our bodies because our cells are functioning at their optimal level. The more youthful genes are turned on, the detox processes are humming along, the immune system is nicely balanced between antibody creation and virus killing and cancer protection. Everything is designed to protect the cells and the organisms in order for you to reproduce.

Because we're performing at our optimal level, we feel like we can get away with abusing our cells: not sleeping well, drinking too much alcohol, lots of emotional stress, eating poorly and not getting adequate nutrients, living a sedentary lifestyle, smoking, environmental toxins in our beauty products, lead in the air or water, mercury fillings, and EMF exposure.

When your cells are younger, they have unlimited resources. The absorptive surfaces of your intestines can get all the nutrients out of any food that you put in. Your body's trash systems are working properly so your lymphatic drainage and liver systems work perfectly. All of this is designed to keep your body running until it's able to reproduce. Once the reproductive and child-raising years are past, all those switches get flipped off inside the cells so that there's not as much reason to preserve your body. It is biology's preservation of the entire species as well as you.

These changes are gradual. Your intestinal absorption isn't as good; your reflexes aren't as quick; your cognitive abilities aren't as sharp; your executive function isn't as rapid. You can't remember the name of something or can't hold lists of things in your head like you once did. These aren't big changes, but overall, you're not able to retain as much information—and it's frustrating. If you take classes again in your forties, it's much more difficult to study for a test and memorize information than it was when you were in your twenties; at the same time, taking classes in your forties is one way to reverse this decline, so give yourself some grace and keep learning! All of it—the detox pathways and immune system functions—have been turned down, because you're past your reproductive years.

Don't Let Your Body Do It Alone

Because there is no true way to completely stop this process, it's important to make the proper lifestyle changes to delay the aging process. Peptides are invaluable for reversing your body's internal shutdown, but they are not a miracle cure. There are still billions of peptides left to be discovered, and we still don't know everything about the ones we have available.

All of those other peptides are doing their job in your body every day. There are several naturally occurring peptides called myokines that are produced when you exercise. An exercising muscle produces these myokines that signal to the rest of the body that everything is okay, this body is a youthful person, and that they need to protect and preserve it. Myokines reignite a lot of those youthful expressions. Doing your part—with fitness, diet, and minimizing environmental toxins—takes a load off of your immune system, so it's not having to deal with that extra stress as we try to turn back the clock on your overall cellular health.

If you haven't led a fit lifestyle, today is the day to seize it. If you are forty years old, you probably have at least forty more years; think of it as having an entire life to do all over again, and now you can do it in a new direction. That is what's most exciting—you can actually make more of an impact at age forty than at age twenty by starting a lifestyle intervention. Taking care of yourself through regular exercise, quitting smoking, and improving sleep directly affects osteoporosis and heart health. When you make healthy lifestyle interventions, your body doesn't have to do everything on its own. No matter how small of an initial change, altering your unhealthy habits is one less thing your body won't have to fight.

Don't think of your health journey in terms of diet culture in which lighter means healthier—because it's not true. Keep away from the scale because building muscle through exercise, and therefore gaining muscle mass and weight, is how we communicate to the body that it is well. As I continue doing weightlifting, I'm finding that my weight is going up. I weigh the most that I have ever weighed in my whole life, but I am also leaner than I've ever been. Yes, even leaner than when I was in my twenties, because I didn't do a lot of resistance exercise back then. I was running, but I had a higher percentage of body fat than I do now. For the same size, my muscle mass is greater, which weighs more than the fat. My friend might loan me a pair of pants that, even though we weigh the same number of pounds on the scale, are too big.

We know that visceral fat is associated with increased mortality in general, particularly from heart, lung, kidney, and liver problems. If we can decrease your visceral fat, we know that we can improve mortality, and that's another critical metric to measure. If you're losing weight but what you're losing is muscle, you're being counterproductive to our entire goal. If your doctor is not paying attention to your muscle mass maintenance when you're trying to lose weight, then you need a new doctor—preferably one trained in cellular medicine.

This Is Not Your Friend's Peptide Therapy

We can't take the same peptides as our friends and expect the same result, because everyone is unique. Although I provide example peptide stacks in this book, those stacks are based on my experience with my individual patients and not you as an individual. I might prescribe a different stack for you than for your best friend with similar disease states, because I'm looking at your unique panel of labs, personal medical history, family history, and environmental toxin exposure history. When your doctor tailors a peptide therapy uniquely for you, you're able to see the best results possible.

Occasionally, we feel like we could use just a little extra skin smoothing and hair luster. These results are possible through the use of peptides, but the results often go beyond basic appearance. Peptide therapy will bring back the spark you've been missing; it can improve how you feel, your energy level, and your quality of sleep. All of that is going to give you confidence, which is a youthful emotional expression. If you are confident, people are attracted to you. Being strong, being energetic, and sleeping well all does that.

This change isn't going to happen overnight, however. The difference between peptides and pharmaceuticals is that peptide therapy usually is going to take two or three months to be effective, whereas most pharmaceuticals have immediate results. Some peptides do work quickly, like a lot of the injectables for joints that can resolve issues within one or two treatments. But many of them require two or three months for the signaling cascade to be reversed. The peptides have to enter the cell, turn back on all of those youthful genes, and express those proteins off of that DNA—and then finally those proteins go and do their job as a youthful cell.

This process takes time. Set a realistic expectation that you will commit to this treatment for a period of time recommended by your provider before making a change, because there might be some needed modifications before you see full results. And, because these changes are so gradual, find a way to mark your progress. Otherwise, you may be discouraged, because the results don't appear obvious although they are working for you. Take before and after photos of your hair regrowth and skin. Do a before and after bioimpedance analysis or DEXA scan of your muscle mass. Wear an Oura ring or other fit tech to measure your sleep, or conduct a before and after polysomnography that helps measure the quality of your sleep. If you stick with it and are patient, I promise the results will be worth the wait.

The New (Old) You is Waiting

After all, wouldn't you prefer to reclaim your youthful expression of these peptides rather than merely surviving? You have so many exciting things to do. You have so much creativity to share with the world. You have mountains to climb, businesses to build, and families to raise. All of that requires more youthful energy, especially because, in today's world, we have more toxins, more environmental issues, and more stressors thrown at us. The twenty-four-hour news cycle alone is enough to raise anyone's blood pressure.

Peptides can be one tool in your health arsenal to restore your body's ability to handle all of these stressors and produce the things that are uniquely yours for the world. Don't let your body hold you back from rising to the challenges you know you can conquer.

If you want to find out more about how peptide therapy can help you age counterclockwise, reach out to Vine Medical and speak to our team.

Website: www.vinemedical.com

Email: info@vinemedical.com

Phone: 404.446.3600

If you're not in the Atlanta area or you find yourself on our waiting list, these sources provide a directory of providers:

- A4M (American Academy of Anti-Aging Medicine)
- IPS (International Peptide Society)
- SSRP (Seeds Scientific Research and Performance)

ENDNOTES

1   Sikirić, P et al. "A new gastric juice peptide, BPC. An overview of the stomach-stress-organoprotection hypothesis and beneficial effects of BPC." *Journal of physiology, Paris* 87, no. 5 (1993): 313-27. PMID: 8298609. https://doi.org/10.1016/0928-4257(93)90038-u.

2   Sikirić, P et al. "A new gastric juice peptide, BPC. An overview of the stomach-stress-organoprotection hypothesis and beneficial effects of BPC." *Journal of physiology, Paris* 87, no. 5 (1993): 313-27. PMID: 8298609. https://doi.org/10.1016/0928-4257(93)90038-u.

3   Sikiric, Predrag et al. "Stable Gastric Pentadecapeptide BPC 157, Robert's Stomach Cytoprotection/Adaptive Cytoprotection/Organoprotection, and Selye's Stress Coping Response: Progress, Achievements, and the Future." *Gut and liver* 14, no. 2 (March 2020): 153-167. PMID: 31158953. https://doi.org/10.5009/gnl18490.

4   Vitaic, S et al. "Nonsteroidal anti-inflammatory drugs-induced failure of lower esophageal and pyloric sphincter and counteraction of sphincters failure with stable gatric pentadecapeptide BPC 157 in rats." *Journal of physiology and pharmacology : an official journal of the Polish Physiological Society* 68, no. 2 (April 2017): 265-272. PMID: 28614776. https://pubmed.ncbi.nlm.nih.gov/28614776/.

5   Vitaic, S et al. "Nonsteroidal anti-inflammatory drugs-induced failure of lower esophageal and pyloric sphincter and counteraction of sphincters failure with stable gatric pentadecapeptide BPC 157 in rats." *Journal of physiology and pharmacology : an official journal of the Polish Physiological Society* 68, no. 2 (April 2017): 265-272. PMID: 28614776. https://pubmed.ncbi.nlm.nih.gov/28614776/.

6   Sun, Xiong, Yao Huang, Ya-Li Zhang, Dan Qiao, and Yan-Cheng Dai. "Research advances of vasoactive intestinal peptide in the pathogenesis of ulcerative colitis by regulating interleukin-10 expression in regulatory B cells." *World journal of gastroenterology* 26, no. 48 (December 2020): 7593-7602. PMID: 33505138. https://doi.org/10.3748/wjg.v26.i48.7593.

7   Greenwood-Van Meerveld, Beverley, Karl Tyler, Ehsan Mohammadi, and Claudio Pietra. "Efficacy of ipamorelin, a ghrelin mimetic, on gastric dysmotility in a rodent model of postoperative ileus." *Journal of experimental pharmacology* 4 (October 2012): 149-55. PMID: 27186127. https://doi.org/10.2147/JEP.S35396.

8   Hoilat, Gilles Jadd et al. "Larazotide acetate for treatment of celiac disease: A systematic review and meta-analysis of randomized controlled trials." *Clinics and research in hepatology and gastroenterology* 46, no. 1 (January 2022): 101782. PMID: 34339872. https://doi.org/10.1016/j.clinre.2021.101782.

9   Leffler, Daniel A et al. "Larazotide acetate for persistent symptoms of celiac disease despite a gluten-free diet: a randomized controlled trial." *Gastroenterology* 148, no. 7 (June 2015): 1311-9.e6. PMID: 25683116. https://doi.org/10.1053/j.gastro.2015.02.008.

10   Di Micco, Simone et al. "*In silico* Analysis Revealed Potential Anti-SARS-CoV-2 Main Protease Activity by the Zonulin Inhibitor Larazotide Acetate." *Frontiers in chemistry* 8 (January 2021): 628609. PMID: 33520943. https://doi.org/10.3389/fchem.2020.628609.

11   Di Micco, Simone et al. "Peptide Derivatives of the Zonulin Inhibitor Larazotide (AT1001) as Potential Anti SARS-CoV-2: Molecular Modelling, Synthesis and Bioactivity Evaluation." *International journal of molecular sciences* 22, no.17 (August 2021): 9427. PMID: 34502335. https://doi.org/10.3390/ijms22179427.

12   Ludwig, Michael D, Anthony P Turel, Ian S Zagon, and Patricia J McLaughlin. "Long-term treatment with low dose naltrexone maintains stable health in patients with multiple sclerosis." *Multiple sclerosis journal - experimental, translational and clinical* 2 (September 2016): 2055217316672242. PMID: 28607740. https://doi.org/10.1177/2055217316672242.

13   Guerrero, Brooke L, and Nancy L Sicotte. "Microglia in Multiple Sclerosis: Friend or Foe?." *Frontiers in immunology* 11 (March 2020): 374. PMID: 32265902. https://doi.org/10.3389/fimmu.2020.00374.

14   Giacomini, Elena et al. "Thymosin-α1 expands deficient IL-10-producing regulatory B cell subsets in relapsing-remitting multiple sclerosis patients." *Multiple sclerosis (Houndmills, Basingstoke, England)* 24, no. 2 (February 2018): 127-139. PMI: 28273784. https://doi.org/10.1177/1352458517695892.

15	Xu, Yunlong et al. "Thymosin Alpha-1 Inhibits Complete Freund's Adjuvant-Induced Pain and Production of Microglia-Mediated Pro-inflammatory Cytokines in Spinal Cord." *Neuroscience bulletin* 35, no. 4 (August 2019): 637-648. PMID: 30790216. https://doi.org/10.1007/s12264-019-00346-z.

16	Matteucci, Claudia et al. "Thymosin Alpha 1 Mitigates Cytokine Storm in Blood Cells From Coronavirus Disease 2019 Patients." *Open forum infectious diseases* 8, no. 1 (December 2020): ofaa588. PMID: 33506065. https://doi.org/10.1093/ofid/ofaa588.

17	Graves, D T, and D L Cochran. "Biologically active mediators: platelet-derived growth factor, monocyte chemoattractant protein-1, and transforming growth factor-beta." *Current opinion in dentistry* 1, no. 6 (December 1991): 809-15. PMID: 1807487; Liu, Yueping et al. "Thymosin Alpha 1 Reduces the Mortality of Severe Coronavirus Disease 2019 by Restoration of Lymphocytopenia and Reversion of Exhausted T Cells." *Clinical infectious diseases : an official publication of the Infectious Diseases Society of America* 71, no. 16 (November 2020): 2150-2157. PMID: 32442287. https://doi.org/10.1093/cid/ciaa630.

18	Dopp, A C, M G Mutchnick, and A L Goldstein. "Thymosin-dependent T-lymphocyte response in inflammatory bowel disease." *Gastroenterology* 79, no. 2 (August 1980): 276-82. PMID: 6967439. https://pubmed.ncbi.nlm.nih.gov/6967439/; Tomazic, V J, Novotny, E A, and Ordonez, J V. "Thymosin alpha 1-induced modulation of cellular responses and functional T-cell subsets in mice with experimental autoimmune thyroiditis." *Cellular immunology* 93, no. 2 (July 1985): 340-9. PMID: 3873993. https://doi.org/10.1016/0008-8749(85)90139-x.

19	Ahmed, Tazeen J, Trinidad Montero-Melendez, Mauro Perretti, and Costantino Pitzalis. "Curbing Inflammation through Endogenous Pathways: Focus on Melanocortin Peptides." *International journal of inflammation* 2013 (May 2013): 985815. PMID: 23738228. https://doi.org/10.1155/2013/985815.

20	Korkmaz, Orhan Tansel et al. "Vasoactive Intestinal Peptide Decreases β-Amyloid Accumulation and Prevents Brain Atrophy in the 5xFAD Mouse Model of Alzheimer's Disease." *Journal of molecular neuroscience : MN* 68, no. 3 (July 2019): 389-396. PMID: 30498985. https://doi.org/10.1007/s12031-018-1226-8.

21	Sun, Xiong, Yao Huang, Ya-Li Zhang, Dan Qiao, and Yan-Cheng Dai. "Research advances of vasoactive intestinal peptide in the pathogenesis of ulcerative colitis by regulating interleukin-10 expression in regulatory B cells." *World journal of gastroenterology* 26, no. 48 (December 2020): 7593-7602. PMID: 33505138. https://doi.org/10.3748/wjg.v26.i48.7593.

22   Youssef, Jihad Georges et al. "The Use of IV Vasoactive Intestinal Peptide (Aviptadil) in Patients With Critical COVID-19 Respiratory Failure: Results of a 60-Day Randomized Controlled Trial." *Critical care medicine* 50, no. 11 (November 2022): 1545-1554. PMID: 36044317. https://doi.org/10.1097/CCM.0000000000005660; Youssef, Jihad Georges et al. "Brief Report: Rapid Clinical Recovery From Critical Coronavirus Disease 2019 With Respiratory Failure in a Pregnant Patient Treated With IV Vasoactive Intestinal Peptide." *Critical care explorations* 4, no. 1 (January 2022): e0607. PMID: 35018346. https://doi.org/10.1097/CCE.0000000000000607.

23   Gong, Yan et al. "Growth hormone alleviates oxidative stress and improves oocyte quality in Chinese women with polycystic ovary syndrome: a randomized controlled trial." *Scientific reports* 10, no. 1 (October 2020): 18769. PMIDD: 33127971. https://doi.org/10.1038/s41598-020-75107-4; Wang, Jianye et al. "Growth hormone protects against ovarian granulosa cell apoptosis: Alleviation oxidative stress and enhancement mitochondrial function." *Reproductive biology* 21, no. 2 (April 2021): 100504. PMID: 33839528. https://doi.org/10.1016/j.repbio.2021.100504.

24   Waseem, Talat, Mark Duxbury, Hiromichi Ito, Stanley W Ashley, and Malcolm K Robinson. "Exogenous ghrelin modulates release of pro-inflammatory and anti-inflammatory cytokines in LPS-stimulated macrophages through distinct signaling pathways." *Surgery* 143, no. 3 (December 2008): 334-42. PMID: 18291254. https://doi.org/10.1016/j.surg.2007.09.039.

25   Catania, Anna. "Neuroprotective actions of melanocortins: a therapeutic opportunity." *Trends in neurosciences* 31, no. 7 (July 2008): 353-60. PMID: 18550183. https://doi.org/10.1016/j.tins.2008.04.002.

26   Goit, Rajesh Kumar, Andrew W Taylor, and Amy Cheuk Yin Lo. "The central melanocortin system as a treatment target for obesity and diabetes: A brief overview." *European journal of pharmacology* 924 (June 2022): 174956. PMID: 35430211. https://doi.org/10.1016/j.ejphar.2022.174956; Fatima, Munazza Tamkeen, Ahmed, Ikhlak, Fakhro, Khalid Adnan, Akil, Ammira Sarah Al-Shabeeb. "Melanocortin-4 receptor complexity in energy homeostasis,obesity and drug

development strategies." *Diabetes, obesity & metabolism* 24, no. 4 (April 2022): 583-598. PMID: 34882941. https://doi.org/10.1111/dom.14618.

27   Galimberti, D et al. "Alpha-MSH peptides inhibit production of nitric oxide and tumor necrosis factor-alpha by microglial cells activated with beta-amyloid and interferon gamma." *Biochemical and biophysical research communications* 263, no. 1 (September 1999): 251-6. PMID: 10486285. https://doi.org/10.1006/bbrc.1999.1276.

28   Kannengiesser, Klaus et al. "Melanocortin-derived tripeptide KPV has anti-inflammatory potential in murine models of inflammatory bowel disease." *Inflammatory bowel diseases* 14, no. 3 (March 2008): 324-31. PMID: 18092346. https://doi.org/10.1002/ibd.20334.

29   Sertié, Rogério Antônio Laurato et al. "Acute growth hormone administration increases myoglobin expression and Glut4 translocation in rat cardiac muscle cells." *Metabolism: clinical and experimental* 63, no. 12 (August 2014): 1499-502. PMID: 25306099. https://doi.org/10.1016/j.metabol.2014.08.012.

30   Poudel, Sher Bahadur et al. "Effects of GH/IGF on the Aging Mitochondria." *Cells* 9, no. 6 (June 2020): 1384. PMID: 32498386. https://doi.org/10.3390/cells9061384.

31   Short, Kevin R et al. "Enhancement of muscle mitochondrial function by growth hormone." *The Journal of clinical endocrinology and metabolism* 93, no. 2 (February 2008): 597-604. PMID: 18000087. https://doi.org/10.1210/jc.2007-1814.

32   Lee, Changhan et al. "The mitochondrial-derived peptide MOTS-c promotes metabolic homeostasis and reduces obesity and insulin resistance." *Cell metabolism* 21, no. 3 (2015): 443-54. PMID: 25738459. https://doi.org/10.1016/j.cmet.2015.02.009.

33   Mohtashami, Zahra et al. "MOTS-c, the Most Recent Mitochondrial Derived Peptide in Human Aging and Age-Related Diseases." *International journal of molecular sciences* 23, no. 19 (October 2022): 11991. PMID: 36233287. https://doi.org/10.3390/ijms231911991.

34   Whitson, Jeremy A et al. "SS-31 and NMN: Two paths to improve metabolism and function in aged hearts." *Aging cell* 19, no. 10 (August 2020): e13213. PMID: 32779818. https://doi.org/10.1111/acel.13213; Campbell, Matthew D et al. "Improving mitochondrial function with SS-31 reverses age-related redox stress and improves exercise tolerance in aged mice." *Free radical biology & medicine* 134 (April 2019): 268-281. PMID: 30597195. https://doi.org/10.1016/j.

freeradbiomed.2018.12.031; Escribano-Lopez, Irene et al. "The mitochondrial antioxidant SS-31 increases SIRT1 levels and ameliorates inflammation, oxidative stress and leukocyte-endothelium interactions in type 2 diabetes." *Scientific reports* 8, no. 1 (October 2018): 15862. PMID: 30367115. https://doi.org/10.1038/s41598-018-34251-8.

35   Cartwright, Claire et al. "Long-term antidepressant use: patient perspectives of benefits and adverse effects." *Patient preference and adherence* 10 (July 2016): 1401-7. PMID: 27528803. https://doi.org/10.2147/PPA.S110632.

36   Zhan, Xinhua, Boryana Stamova, and Frank R Sharp. "Lipopolysaccharide Associates with Amyloid Plaques, Neurons and Oligodendrocytes in Alzheimer's Disease Brain: A Review." *Frontiers in aging neuroscience* 10 (February 2018): 42. PMID: 29520228. https://doi.org/10.3389/fnagi.2018.00042.

37   Andrianne, Y et al. "External fixation pin: an in vitro general investigation." *Orthopedics* 10, no. 11 (November 1987): 1507-16. PMID: 3684796. https://pubmed.ncbi.nlm.nih.gov/3684796/.

38   Gauthier, Serge et al. "Cerebrolysin in mild-to-moderate Alzheimer's disease: a meta-analysis of randomized controlled clinical trials." *Dementia and geriatric cognitive disorders* 39, no. 5-6 (March 2015): 332-47. PMID: 25832905. https://doi.org/10.1159/000377672; Gavrilova, Svetlana I, and Anton Alvarez. "Cerebrolysin in the therapy of mild cognitive impairment and dementia due to Alzheimer's disease: 30 years of clinical use." *Medicinal research reviews* 41, no. 5 (September 2021): 2775-2803. PMID: 32808294. https://doi.org/10.1002/med.21722; Gharagozli, K et al. "Efficacy and safety of Cerebrolysin treatment in early recovery after acute ischemic stroke: a randomized, placebo-controlled, double-blinded, multicenter clinical trial." *Journal of medicine and life* 10, no. 3 (July-September 2017): 153-160. PMID: 29075343. https://pubmed.ncbi.nlm.nih.gov/29075343/; Ozkizilcik, Asya et al. "Nanodelivery of cerebrolysin reduces pathophysiology of Parkinson's disease." *Progress in brain research* 245 (April 2019): 201-246. PMID: 30961868. https://doi.org/10.1016/bs.pbr.2019.03.014; Khabirov, F A et al. "Primenenie tserebrolizina u bol'nykh rasseyannym sklerozom v stadii regressa obostreniya" [Effect of cerebrolysin on remyelination processes in multiple sclerosis patients in stage of relapse regression]. *Zhurnal nevrologii i psikhiatrii imeni S.S. Korsakova* 116, no. 12 (2016): 48-53. PMID: 28139626, https://doi.org/10.17116/jnevro201611612148-53; Mureşanu, Ioana Anamaria et al. "The Effect of Cerebrolysin on Anx-

iety, Depression, and Cognition in Moderate and Severe Traumatic Brain Injury Patients: A CAPTAIN II Retrospective Trial Analysis." *Medicina (Kaunas, Lithuania)* 58, no. 5 (May 2022): 648. PMID: 35630065. https://doi.org/10.3390/medicina58050648; Ghaffarpasand, Fariborz et al. "Effects of cerebrolysin on functional outcome of patients with traumatic brain injury: a systematic review and meta-analysis." *Neuropsychiatric disease and treatment* 15 (December 2018): 127-135. PMID: 30643411. https://doi.org/10.2147/NDT.S186865; Chutko, L S et al. "Narusheniia kognitivnogo kontrolia pri sindrome defitsita vnimaniia u vzroslykh" [Cognitive control impairment in adult with attention deficit/hyperactivity disorder]. *Zhurnal nevrologii i psikhiatrii imeni S.S. Korsakova* 118, no. 12 (2018): 31-35. PMID: 30698557. https://doi.org/10.17116/jnevro201811812131.

39   Mahmoudi, Javad et al. "Cerebrolysin attenuates hyperalgesia, photophobia, and neuroinflammation in a nitroglycerin-induced migraine model in rats." *Brain research bulletin* 140 (June 2018): 197-204. PMID: 29752991. https://doi.org/10.1016/j.brainresbull.2018.05.008; Morales-Medina, Julio C et al. "Cerebrolysin improves peripheral inflammatory pain: Sex differences in two models of acute and chronic mechanical hypersensitivity." *Drug development research* 80, no. 4 (June 2019): 513-518. PMID: 30908710. https://doi.org/10.1002/ddr.21528.

40   Sun, Xiaojin et al. "AngIV-Analog Dihexa Rescues Cognitive Impairment and Recovers Memory in the APP/PS1 Mouse via the PI3K/AKT Signaling Pathway." *Brain sciences* 11, no. 11 (November 2021): 1487. PMID: 34827486. https://doi.org/10.3390/brainsci11111487; Weiss, Jessica B et al. "Stem cell, Granulocyte-Colony Stimulating Factor and/or Dihexa to promote limb function recovery in a rat sciatic nerve damage-repair model: Experimental animal studies." *Annals of medicine and surgery (2012)* 71 (October 2021): 102917. PMID: 34703584. https://doi.org/10.1016/j.amsu.2021.102917; Desole, Claudia et al. "HGF and MET: From Brain Development to Neurological Disorders." *Frontiers in cell and developmental biology* 9 (June 2021): 683609. PMID: 34179015. https://doi.org10.3389/fcell.2021.683609.

41   Desole, Claudia et al. "HGF and MET: From Brain Development to Neurological Disorders." *Frontiers in cell and developmental biology* 9 (June 2021): 683609. PMID: 25187433. https://doi.org/10.3389/fcell.2021.683609; Wright, John W et al. "The development of small molecule angiotensin IV analogs to treat Alzheimer's and Parkinson's

diseases." *Progress in neurobiology* 125 (February 2015): 26-46. PMID: 25455861. https://doi.org/10.1016/j.pneurobio.2014.11.004.

42   Lugenbiel, Patrick et al. "TREK-1 ($K_{2P}2.1$) K^+ channels are suppressed in patients with atrial fibrillation and heart failure and provide therapeutic targets for rhythm control." *Basic research in cardiology* 112, no. 1 (January 2017): 8. PMID: 28005193. https://doi.org/10.1007/s00395-016-0597-7; Djillani, Alaeddine et al. "Role of TREK-1 in Health and Disease, Focus on the Central Nervous System." *Frontiers in pharmacology* 10 (April 2019): 379. PMID: 31031627. https://doi.org/10.3389/fphar.2019.00379; Fang, Yongkang et al. "Deficiency of TREK-1 potassium channel exacerbates blood-brain barrier damage and neuroinflammation after intracerebral hemorrhage in mice." *Journal of neuroinflammation* 16, no. 1 (May 2019): 96. PMID: 31072336. https://doi.org/10.1186/s12974-019-1485-5.

43   Chez, Michael G et al. "Double-blind, placebo-controlled study of L-carnosine supplementation in children with autistic spectrum disorders." *Journal of child neurology* 17, no. 11 (November 2002): 833-7. PMID: 12585724. https://doi.org/10.1177/08830738020170111 501; Hajizadeh-Zaker, Reihaneh et al. "l-Carnosine As an Adjunctive Therapy to Risperidone in Children with Autistic Disorder: A Randomized, Double-Blind, Placebo-Controlled Trial." *Journal of child and adolescent psychopharmacology* 28, no. 1 (February 2018): 74-81. PMID: 29027815. https://doi.org/10.1089/cap.2017.0026.

44   Eremin, K O et al. "Effects of Semax on dopaminergic and serotoninergic systems of the brain." *Doklady biological sciences : proceedings of the Academy of Sciences of the USSR, Biological sciences sections* 394 (January-February 2004): 1-3. PMID: 15088389. https://doi.org/10.1023/b:dobs.0000017114.24474.40.

45   Samotrueva, M A et al. "Experimental Substantiation of Application of Semax as a Modulator of Immune Reaction on the Model of "Social" Stress." *Bulletin of experimental biology and medicine* 166, no. 6 (April 2019): 754-758. PMID: 31028579. https://doi.org/10.1007/s10517-019-04434-y.

46   Filippenkov, Ivan B et al. "Novel Insights into the Protective Properties of $ACTH_{(4-7)}$PGP (Semax) Peptide at the Transcriptome Level Following Cerebral Ischaemia-Reperfusion in Rats." *Genes* 11, no. 6 (June 2020): 681. PMID: 32580520. https://doi.org/10.3390/genes11060681.

47   Tsai, Shih-Jen. "Semax, an analogue of adrenocorticotropin (4-10), is a potential agent for the treatment of attention-deficit hyperactivity disorder and Rett syndrome." *Medical hypotheses* 68, no. 5 (2007): 1144-6. PMID: 16996699. https://doi.org/10.1016/j.mehy.2006.07.017.

48   Sokolov, O Yu, N K Meshavkin, N V Kost, and A A Zozulya. "Effects of Selank on behavioral reactions and activities of plasma enkephalin-degrading enzymes in mice with different phenotypes of emotional and stress reactions." *Bulletin of experimental biology and medicine* 133, no. 2 (February 2002): 133-5. PMID: 12432865. https://doi.org/10.1023/a:1015582302311.

49   Volkova, Anastasiya et al. "Selank Administration Affects the Expression of Some Genes Involved in GABAergic Neurotransmission." *Frontiers in pharmacology* 7 (February 2016): 31. PMID: 26924987. https://doi.org/10.3389/fphar.2016.00031.

50   Tudor, Mario et al. "Traumatic brain injury in mice and pentadecapeptide BPC 157 effect." *Regulatory peptides* 160, no. 1-3 (February 2010): 26-32. PMID: 19931318. https://doi.org/10.1016/j.regpep.2009.11.012.

51   Scoccianti, Chiara et al. "Female breast cancer and alcohol consumption: a review of the literature." *American journal of preventive medicine* 46, no. 3 Suppl 1 (March 2014): S16-25. PMID: 24512927. https://doi.org/10.1016/j.amepre.2013.10.031.

52   Dieli-Conwright, Christina M et al. "Effect of aerobic and resistance exercise on the mitochondrial peptide MOTS-c in Hispanic and Non-Hispanic White breast cancer survivors." *Scientific reports* 11, no. 1 (August 2021): 16916. PMID: 34413391. https://doi.org/10.1038/s41598-021-96419-z.

53   Baggio, Laurie L, and Daniel J Drucker. "Biology of incretins: GLP-1 and GIP." *Gastroenterology* 132, no. 6 (May 2007): 2131-57. PMID: 17498508. https://doi.org/10.1053/j.gastro.2007.03.054.

54   Iepsen, Eva W et al. "GLP-1 Receptor Agonist Treatment Increases Bone Formation and Prevents Bone Loss in Weight-Reduced Obese Women." *The Journal of clinical endocrinology and metabolism* 100, no. 8 (August 2015): 2909-17. PMID: 26043228. https://doi.org/10.1210/jc.2015-1176; Salamun, Vesna, Mojca Jensterle, Andrej Janez, and Eda Vrtacnik Bokal. "Liraglutide increases IVF pregnancy rates in obese PCOS women with poor response to first-line re-

productive treatments: a pilot randomized study." *European journal of endocrinology* 179, no. 1 (July 2018): 1-11. PMID: 29703793. https://doi.org/10.1530/EJE-18-0175; Pi-Sunyer, Xavier et al. "A Randomized, Controlled Trial of 3.0 mg of Liraglutide in Weight Management." *The New England journal of medicine* 373, no. 1 (July 2015): 11-22. PMID: 26132939. https://doi.org/10.1056/NEJMoa1411892; Górriz, José Luis et al. "GLP-1 Receptor Agonists and Diabetic Kidney Disease: A Call of Attention to Nephrologists." *Journal of clinical medicine* 9, no. 4 (March 2020): 947. PMID: 32235471. https://doi.org/10.3390/jcm9040947; Mantovani, Alessandro et al. "Glucagon-Like Peptide-1 Receptor Agonists for Treatment of Nonalcoholic Fatty Liver Disease and Nonalcoholic Steatohepatitis: An Updated Meta-Analysis of Randomized Controlled Trials." *Metabolites* 11, no. 2 (January 2021): 73. PMID: 33513761. https://doi.org/10.3390/metabo11020073; Sattar, Naveed et al. "Cardiovascular, mortality, and kidney outcomes with GLP-1 receptor agonists in patients with type 2 diabetes: a systematic review and meta-analysis of randomised trials." *The lancet. Diabetes & endocrinology* 9, no. 10 (October 2021): 653-662. PMID: 34425083. https://doi.org/10.1016/S2213-8587(21)00203-5; Meurot, C et al. "Liraglutide, a glucagon-like peptide 1 receptor agonist, exerts analgesic, anti-inflammatory and anti-degradative actions in osteoarthritis." *Scientific reports* 12, no. 1 (January 2022): 1567. PMID: 35091584. https://doi.org/10.1038/s41598-022-05323-7.

55   Tulipano, Giovanni, Valeria Sibilia, Anna Maria Caroli, and Daniela Cocchi. "Whey proteins as source of dipeptidyl dipeptidase IV (dipeptidyl peptidase-4) inhibitors." *Peptides* 32, no. 4 (April 2011): 835-8. PMID: 21256171. https://doi.org/10.1016/j.peptides.2011.01.002.

56   Gejl, Michael et al. "In Alzheimer's Disease, 6-Month Treatment with GLP-1 Analog Prevents Decline of Brain Glucose Metabolism: Randomized, Placebo-Controlled, Double-Blind Clinical Trial." *Frontiers in aging neuroscience* 8 (May 2016): 108. PMID:27252647. https://do.org/:10.3389/fnagi.2016.00108.

57   Baggio, Laurie L, and Daniel J Drucker. "Biology of incretins: GLP-1 and GIP." *Gastroenterology* 132, no. 6 (May 2007): 2131-57. PMID: 17498508. https://doi.org/10.1053/j.gastro.2007.03.054.

58   Jastreboff, Ania M et al. "Tirzepatide Once Weekly for the Treatment of Obesity." *The New England journal of medicine* 387, no. 3 (July 2022): 205-216. PMID: 35658024. https://doi.org/10.1056/NEJMoa2206038.

59   Ng, F M et al. "Metabolic studies of a synthetic lipolytic domain (AOD9604) of human growth hormone." *Hormone research* 53, no. 6 (2000): 274-8. PMID: 11146367. https://doi.org/10.1159/000053183.

60   Choi, Yang-Ho et al. "MTII administered peripherally reduces fat without invoking apoptosis in rats." *Physiology & behavior* 79, no. 2 (July 2003): 331-7. PMID: 12834806. https://doi.org/10.1016/s0031-9384(03)00118-5.

61   Lee, Changhan et al. "The mitochondrial-derived peptide MOTS-c promotes metabolic homeostasis and reduces obesity and insulin resistance." *Cell metabolism* 21, no. 3 (March 2015): 443-54. https://doi.org/10.1016/j.cmet.2015.02.009; Lu, Huanyu et al. "MOTS-c peptide regulates adipose homeostasis to prevent ovariectomy-induced metabolic dysfunction." *Journal of molecular medicine (Berlin, Germany)* 97, no. 4 (April 2019): 473-485. PMID: 30725119. https://doi.org/10.1007/s00109-018-01738-w.

62   Kerem, Liya, and Elizabeth A Lawson. "The Effects of Oxytocin on Appetite Regulation, Food Intake and Metabolism in Humans." *International journal of molecular sciences* 22, no. 14 (July 2021): 7737. PMID: 34299356. https://doi:10.3390/ijms22147737; Lawson, Elizabeth A. "The effects of oxytocin on eating behaviour and metabolism in humans." *Nature reviews. Endocrinology* 13, no. 12 (December 2017): 700-709. PMID: 28960210. https://doi.org/10.1038/nrendo.2017.115; Zhang, Hai et al. "Treatment of obesity and diabetes using oxytocin or analogs in patients and mouse models." *PloS one* 8, no. 5 (May 2013): e61477. PMID: 23700406. https://doi.org/10.1371/journal.pone.0061477.

63   Vijayakumar, Archana et al. "Biological effects of growth hormone on carbohydrate and lipid metabolism." *Growth hormone & IGF research : official journal of the Growth Hormone Research Society and the International IGF Research Society* 20, no. 1 (February 2010): 1-7. PMID: 19800274. https://doi.org/10.1016/j.ghir.2009.09.002.

64   Scacchi, M, A I Pincelli, and F Cavagnini. "Growth hormone in obesity." *International journal of obesity and related metabolic disorders : journal of the International Association for the Study of Obesity* 23, no. 3 (March 1999): 260-71. PMID: 10193871. https://doi.org/10.1038/sj.ijo.0800807.

65   Sivakumar, T, Oj Mechanic, D A Fehmie, and Bt Paul. "Growth hormone axis treatments for HIV-associated lipodystrophy: a systematic review of placebo-controlled trials." *HIV medicine* 12,

no. 8 (2011): 453-62. PMID: 21265979. https://doi.org/10.1111/j.1468-1293.2010.00906.x.

66   Gatti, R, E F De Palo, G Antonelli, and P Spinella. "IGF-I/IGFBP system: metabolism outline and physical exercise." *Journal of endocrinological investigation* 35, no. 7 (July 2012): 699-707. PMID: 2274057. https://doi.org/10.3275/8456.

67   Gehmert, Sebastian et al. "Adipose tissue-derived stem cell secreted IGF-1 protects myoblasts from the negative effect of myostatin." *BioMed research international* 2014 (2014): 129048. PMID: 24575400. https://doi.org/10.1155/2014/129048.

68   Matheny, Ronald W Jr, Bradley C Nindl, and Martin L Adamoo. "Minireview: Mechano-growth factor: a putative product of IGF-I gene expression involved in tissue repair and regeneration." *Endocrinology* 151, no. 3 (March 2010): 865-75. PMID: 20130113. https://doi.org/10.1210/en.2009-1217.

69   Sha, Yongqiang et al. "Mechano Growth Factor Accelerates ACL Repair and Improves Cell Mobility of Mechanically Injured Human ACL Fibroblasts by Targeting Rac1-PAK1/2 and RhoA-ROCK1 Pathways." *International journal of molecular sciences* 23, no. 8 (April 2022): 4331. PMID: 35457148. https://doi.org/10.3390/ijms23084331.

70   Hatagami Marques, Júlia et al. "Intragenic Deletion in the LIFR Gene in a Long-Term Survivor with Stüve-Wiedemann Syndrome." *Molecular syndromology* 6, no. 2 (July 2015): 87-90. PMID: 26279654. https://doi.org/10.1159/000407418.

71   Kwon, Dong Rak, and Gi Young Park. "Effect of Intra-articular Injection of AOD9604 with or without Hyaluronic Acid in Rabbit Osteoarthritis Model." *Annals of clinical and laboratory science* 45, no. 4 (Summer 2015): 426-32. PMID: 26275694. https://pubmed.ncbi.nlm.nih.gov/26275694/.

72   Cerovecki, Tomislav et al. "Pentadecapeptide BPC 157 (PL 14736) improves ligament healing in the rat." *Journal of orthopaedic research : official publication of the Orthopaedic Research Society* 28, no. 9 (September 2010): 1155-61. PMID: 20225319. https://doi.org/10.1002/jor.21107.

73   Lee, Edwin, and Blake Padgett. "Intra-Articular Injection of BPC 157 for Multiple Types of Knee Pain." *Alternative therapies in health and medicine* 27, no. 4 (July 2021): 8-13. PMID: 34324435. https://pubmed.ncbi.nlm.nih.gov/34324435/; Pevec, Danira et al. "Impact of

pentadecapeptide BPC 157 on muscle healing impaired by systemic corticosteroid application." *Medical science monitor : international medical journal of experimental and clinical research* 16, no. 3 (March 2010): BR81-88. PMID: 20190676. https://pubmed.ncbi.nlm.nih.gov/20190676/.

74   Kozlovskii, I I, and N D Danchev. "The optimizing action of the synthetic peptide Selank on a conditioned active avoidance reflex in rats." *Neuroscience and behavioral physiology* 33, no. 7 (September 2003): 639-43. PMID: 14552529. https://doi.org/10.1023/a:1024444321191.

75   Leonidovna, Yasenyavskaya A et al. "The Influence of Selank on the Level of Cytokines Under the Conditions of "Social" Stress." *Current reviews in clinical and experimental pharmacology* 16, no. 2 (2021): 162-167. PMID: 32621722. https://doi.org/10.2174/1574884715666200704152810.

76   Dolotov, Oleg V et al. "Semax, an analog of ACTH(4-10) with cognitive effects, regulates BDNF and trkB expression in the rat hippocampus." *Brain research* 1117, no. 1 (October 2006): 54-60. PMID: 16996037. https://doi.org/10.1016/j.brainres.2006.07.108.

77   Filippenkov, Ivan B et al. "Antistress Action of Melanocortin Derivatives Associated with Correction of Gene Expression Patterns in the Hippocampus of Male Rats Following Acute Stress." *International journal of molecular sciences* 22, no. 18 (September 2021): 10054. PMID: 34576218. https://doi.org/10.3390/ijms221810054.

78   Hyatt, Jon-Philippe K. "MOTS-c increases in skeletal muscle following long-term physical activity and improves acute exercise performance after a single dose." *Physiological reports* 10, no. 13 (July 2022): e15377. PMID: 35808870. https://doi.org/10.14814/phy2.15377.

79   Reynolds, Joseph C et al. "MOTS-c is an exercise-induced mitochondrial-encoded regulator of age-dependent physical decline and muscle homeostasis." *Nature communications* 12, no. 1 (January 2021): 470. PMMID: 33473109. https://doi.org/10.1038/s41467-020-20790-0.

80   Meurot, C et al. "Liraglutide, a glucagon-like peptide 1 receptor agonist, exerts analgesic, anti-inflammatory and anti-degradative actions in osteoarthritis." *Scientific reports* 12, no. 1 (January 2022): 1567. PMID: 35091584. https://doi.org/10.1038/s41598-022-05323-7; Jeon, Ja Young et al. "GLP1 improves palmitateinduced insulin resistance in human skeletal muscle via SIRT1 activity." *International jour-*

nal of molecular medicine 44, no. 3 (September 2019): 1161-1171. PMID: 31524229. https://doi.org/10.3892/ijmm.2019.4272.

81   Weiss, Jessica B et al. "Stem cell, Granulocyte-Colony Stimulating Factor and/or Dihexa to promote limb function recovery in a rat sciatic nerve damage-repair model: Experimental animal studies." *Annals of medicine and surgery (2012)* 71 (October 2021): 102917. PMID: 34703584. https://doi.org/10.1016/j.amsu.2021.102917.

82   McCormack, Shana E, James E Blevins, and Elizabeth A Lawson. "Metabolic Effects of Oxytocin." *Endocrine reviews* 41, no. 2 (April 2020): 121-145. PMID: 31803919. https://doi.org/10.1210/endrev/bnz012.

83   Ferrero, Stephanie, Ez-Zoubir Amri, and Christian Hubert Roux. "Relationship between Oxytocin and Osteoarthritis: Hope or Despair?." *International journal of molecular sciences* 22, no. 21 (October 2021): 11784. PMID: 34769215. https://doi.org/10.3390/ijms222111784.

84   Meinhardt, Udo et al. "The effects of growth hormone on body composition and physical performance in recreational athletes: a randomized trial." *Annals of internal medicine* 152, no. 9 (May 2010): 568-77. PMID: 20439575. https://doi.org/10.7326/0003-4819-152-9-201005040-00007; Guha, Nishan et al. "The Effects of Recombinant Human Insulin-Like Growth Factor-I/Insulin-Like Growth Factor Binding Protein-3 Administration on Body Composition and Physical Fitness in Recreational Athletes." *The Journal of clinical endocrinology and metabolism* 100, no. 8 (August 2015): 3126-31. PMID: 26046967. https://doi.org/10.1210/jc.2015-1996.

85   Eklund, Emma et al. "IGF-I and IGFBP-1 in Relation to Body Composition and Physical Performance in Female Olympic Athletes." *Frontiers in endocrinology* 12 (August 2021): 708421. PMID: 334484121. https://doi.org/10.3389/fendo.2021.708421.

86   Bramnert, Margareta et al. "Growth hormone replacement therapy induces insulin resistance by activating the glucose-fatty acid cycle." *The Journal of clinical endocrinology and metabolism* 88, no. 4 (April 2003): 1455-63. PMID: 12679422. https://doi.org/10.1210/jc.2002-020542.

87   Blagosklonny, Mikhail V. "Fasting and rapamycin: diabetes versus benevolent glucose intolerance." *Cell death & disease* 10, no.8

(August 2019): 607. PMID: 31406105. https://doi.org/10.1038/s41419-019-1822-8.

88   Bowers, C Y et al. "Growth hormone (GH)-releasing peptide stimulates GH release in normal men and acts synergistically with GH-releasing hormone." *The Journal of clinical endocrinology and metabolism* 70, no. 4 (April 1990): 975-82. PMID: 2108187. https://doi.org/10.1210/jcem-70-4-975.

89   Vittone, J et al. "Effects of single nightly injections of growth hormone-releasing hormone (GHRH 1-29) in healthy elderly men." *Metabolism: clinical and experimental* 46, no. 1 (January 1997): 89-96. PMID: 9005976. https://doi.org/10.1016/s0026-0495(97)90174-8; Steiger, A et al. "Growth hormone-releasing hormone (GHRH)-induced effects on sleep EEG and nocturnal secretion of growth hormone, cortisol and ACTH in patients with major depression." *Journal of psychiatric research* 28, no. 3 (May-June 1994): 225-38. PMID: 7932284. https://doi.org/10.1016/0022-3956(94)90008-6.

90   Boström, Pontus et al. "A PGC1-α-dependent myokine that drives brown-fat-like development of white fat and thermogenesis." *Nature* 481, no. 7382 (January 2012): 463-8. PMID: 22237023. https://doi.org/10.1038/nature10777.

91   Rana, Karan S et al. "Plasma irisin levels predict telomere length in healthy adults." *Age (Dordrecht, Netherlands)* 36, no. 2 (April 2014): 995-1001. PMID: 24469890. https://doi.org/10.1007/s11357-014-9620-9.

92   Liu, Shiqiang et al. "Role of irisin in physiology and pathology." *Frontiers in endocrinology* 13 (September 2022): 962968. PMID: 36225200. https://doi.org/10.3389/fendo.2022.962968.

93   Bi, Jianbin et al. "Irisin alleviates liver ischemia-reperfusion injury by inhibiting excessive mitochondrial fission, promoting mitochondrial biogenesis and decreasing oxidative stress." *Redox biology* 20 (January 2019): 296-306. PMID: 30388684. https://doi.org/10.1016/j.redox.2018.10.019; Bi, Jianbin et al. "Irisin reverses intestinal epithelial barrier dysfunction during intestinal injury via binding to the integrin αVβ5 receptor." *Journal of cellular and molecular medicine* 24, no. 1 (January 2020): 996-1009. PMID: 31701659. https://doi.org/10.1111/jcmm.14811.

94   Liu, Yaqiang et al. "The Neuroprotective Effect of Irisin in Ischemic Stroke." *Frontiers in aging neuroscience* 12 (December 2020):

588958. PMID: 33414714. https://doi.org/10.3389/fnagi.2020.588958; Uysal, Nazan et al. "Regular aerobic exercise correlates with reduced anxiety and incresed levels of irisin in brain and white adipose tissue." *Neuroscience letters* 676 (May 2018): 92-97. PMID: 29655944. https://doi.org/10.1016/j.neulet.2018.04.023.

95   Huh, J Y, F Dincer, E Mesfum, and C S Mantzoros. "Irisin stimulates muscle growth-related genes and regulates adipocyte differentiation and metabolism in humans." *International journal of obesity (2005)* 38, no. 12 (December 2014): 1538-44. PMID: 24614098. https://doi.org/10.1038/ijo.2014.42.

96   Colaianni, G et al. "Crosstalk Between Muscle and Bone Via the Muscle-Myokine Irisin." *Current osteoporosis reports* 14, no. 4 (August 2016): 132-7. PMID: 27299471. https://doi.org/10.1007/s11914-016-0313-4.

97   Wang, Feng-Sheng et al. "Irisin Mitigates Oxidative Stress, Chondrocyte Dysfunction and Osteoarthritis Development through Regulating Mitochondrial Integrity and Autophagy." *Antioxidants (Basel, Switzerland)* 9, no. 9 (September 2020): 810. PMID: 32882839. https://doi.org/10.3390/antiox9090810.

98   Erren, T C et al. "Sleep and cancer: Synthesis of experimental data and meta-analyses of cancer incidence among some 1,500,000 study individuals in 13 countries." *Chronobiology international* 33, no. 4 (2016): 325-50. PMID: 27003385. https://doi.org/10.3109/07420528.2016.1149486; Thomson, Cynthia A et al. "Relationship between sleep quality and quantity and weight loss in women participating in a weight-loss intervention trial." *Obesity (Silver Spring, Md.)* 20, no. 7 (July 2012): 1419-25. PMID: 22402738. https://doi.org/10.1038/oby.2012.62; Lao, Xiang Qian et al. "Sleep Quality, Sleep Duration, and the Risk of Coronary Heart Disease: A Prospective Cohort Study With 60,586 Adults." *Journal of clinical sleep medicine : JCSM : official publication of the American Academy of Sleep Medicine* 14, no. 1 (January 2018): 109-117. PMID: 29198294. https://doi.org/10.5664/jcsm.6894.

99   Bes, F, W Hofman, J Schuur, and C Van Boxtel. "Effects of delta sleep-inducing peptide on sleep of chronic insomniac patients. A double-blind study." *Neuropsychobiology* 26, no. 4 (1992): 193-7. PMID: 1299794. https://doi.org/10.1159/000118919.

100   Tukhovskaya, Elena A et al. "DSIP-Like KND Peptide Reduces Brain Infarction in C57Bl/6 and Reduces Myocardial Infarction in SD Rats When Administered during Reperfusion." *Biomedicines*

9, no. 4 (April 2021): 407. PMID: 33918965. https://doi.org/10.3390/biomedicines9040407.

101   Khavinson, V et al. "Synthetic tetrapeptide epitalon restores disturbed neuroendocrine regulation in senescent monkeys." *Neuro endocrinology letters* 22, no. 4 (August 2001): 251-4. PMID: 11524632. https://pubmed.ncbi.nlm.nih.gov/11524632/.

102   Jain, Vivek et al. "Benefits of oxytocin administration in obstructive sleep apnea." *American journal of physiology. Lung cellular and molecular physiology* 313, no. 5 (November 2017): L825-L833. PMID: 28798255. https://doi.org/10.1152/ajplung.00206.2017.

103   Jain, Vivek et al. "Intranasal oxytocin increases respiratory rate and reduces obstructive event duration and oxygen desaturation in obstructive sleep apnea patients: a randomized double blinded placebo controlled study." *Sleep medicine* 74 (October 2020): 242-247. PMID: 328620007. https://doi.org/10.1016/j.sleep.2020.05.034.

104   Koplik, E V et al. "Blood albumin in the mechanisms of individual resistance of rats to emotional stress." *Neuroscience and behavioral physiology* 33, no. 8 (October 2003): 827-32. PMID: 14636000. https://doi.org/10.1023/a:1025109717945.

105   Obal, Ferenc Jr, and James M Krueger. "GHRH and sleep." *Sleep medicine reviews* 8, no. 5 (October 2004): 367-77. PMID: 15336237. https://doi.org/10.1016/j.smrv.2004.03.005; Peterfi, Zoltan, Dennis McGinty, Erzsebet Sarai, and Ronald Szymusiak. "Growth hormone-releasing hormone activates sleep regulatory neurons of the rat preoptic hypothalamus." *American journal of physiology. Regulatory, integrative and comparative physiology* 298, no. 1 (January 2010): R147-56. PMID: 198899861. https://doi.org/10.1152/ajpregu.00494.2009.

106   Toro, Carlos A et al. "Boldine modulates glial transcription and functional recovery in a murine model of contusion spinal cord injury." *bioRxiv* Preprint (February 2023). PMID: 36824813. https://doi.org/ 10.1101/2023.02.15.528337.

107   Prospéro-Garcia, O, M Morales, G Arankowsky-Sandoval, and R Drucker-Colin. "Vasoactive intestinal polypeptide (VIP) and cerebrospinal fluid (CSF) of sleep-deprived cats restores REM sleep in insomniac recipients." *Brain research* 385, no. 1 (October 1986): 169-73. PMID: 2945620. https://doi.org/10.1016/0006-8993(86)91561-1; Murck, H et al. "VIP decelerates non-REM-REM cycles and modulates hormone secretion during sleep in men." *The American journal of phys-*

iology 271, no. 4 Pt 2 (October 1996): R905-11. PMID: 8897980. https://doi.org/10.1152/ajpregu.1996.271.4.R905.

108   Hu, Wang-Ping, Jia-Da Li, Christopher S Colwell, and Qun-Yong Zhou. "Decreased REM sleep and altered circadian sleep regulation in mice lacking vasoactive intestinal polypeptide." *Sleep* 34, no. 1 (January 2011): 49-56. PMID: 21203371. https://doi.org/10.1093/sleep/34.1.49.

109   Kumar, Naina, and Amit Kant Singh. "Trends of male factor infertility, an important cause of infertility: A review of literature." *Journal of human reproductive sciences* 8, no. 4 (October-December 2015): 191-6. PMID: 26752853. https://doi.org/10.4103/0974-1208.170370.

110   Wilcox, A J et al. "Incidence of early loss of pregnancy." *The New England journal of medicine* 319, no. 4 (July 1988): 189-94. PMID: 3393170. https://doi.org/10.1056/NEJM198807283190401.

111   Lamceva, Jelizaveta, Romans Uljanovs, and Ilze Strumfa. "The Main Theories on the Pathogenesis of Endometriosis." *International journal of molecular sciences* 24, no. 5 (February 2023): 4254. PMID: 36901685. https://doi.org/10.3390/ijms24054254.

112   Ding, Kai, Fei Hua, and Wenge Ding. "Gut Microbiome and Osteoporosis." *Aging and disease* 11, no. 2 (March 2020): 438-447. PMID: 32257552. https://doi.org/10.14336/AD.2019.0523.

113   Fiatarone, M A et al. "High-intensity strength training in nonagenarians. Effects on skeletal muscle." *JAMA* 263, no. 22 (June 1990): 3029-34. PMID: 2342214. https://pubmed.ncbi.nlm.nih.gov/2342214/.

114   Novaira, Horacio J et al. "Disrupted kisspeptin signaling in GnRH neurons leads to hypogonadotrophic hypogonadism." *Molecular endocrinology (Baltimore, Md.)* 28, no. 2 (2014): 225-38. PMID: 24422632. https://doi.org/10.1210/me.2013-1319.

115   Abbara, Ali et al. "A second dose of kisspeptin-54 improves oocyte maturation in women at high risk of ovarian hyperstimulation syndrome: a Phase 2 randomized controlled trial." *Human reproduction (Oxford, England)* 32, no. 9 (September 2017): 1915-1924. PMID: 28854728. https://doi.org/10.1093/humrep/dex253; Akkaya, Hatice, Ertugrul Kilic, Signem Eyuboglu Dinc, and Bayram Yilmaz. "Postacute effects of kisspeptin-10 on neuronal injury induced by L-methionine in rats." *Journal of biochemical and molecular toxicology* 28, no. 8 (August 2014): 373-7. PMID: 24863683. https://doi.org/10.1002/jbt.21573; Akad, Mona et al. "Kisspeptin Serum Levels in Patients with Endome-

triosis, New Research Pathways Regarding Female Infertility." *Maedica* 17, no. 3 (September 2022): 557-560. PMID: 36540601. https://doi.org/10.26574/maedica.2022.17.3.557.

116   Salamun, Vesna, Mojca Jensterle, Andrej Janez, and Eda Vrtacnik Bokal. "Liraglutide increases IVF pregnancy rates in obese PCOS women with poor response to first-line reproductive treatments: a pilot randomized study." *European journal of endocrinology* 179, no. 1 (July 2018): 1-11. PMID: 29703793. https://doi.org/10.1530/EJE-18-0175; Cena, Hellas, Luca Chiovato, and Rossella E Nappi. "Obesity, Polycystic Ovary Syndrome, and Infertility: A New Avenue for GLP-1 Receptor Agonists." *The Journal of clinical endocrinology and metabolism* 105, no. 8 (August 2020): e2695–e2709. PMID: 32442310. https://doi.org/10.1210/clinem/dgaa285.

117   Hart, Roger J. "Use of Growth Hormone in the IVF Treatment of Women With Poor Ovarian Reserve." *Frontiers in endocrinology* 10 (July 2019): 500. PMID: 31396160. https://doi.org/10.3389/fendo.2019.00500.

118   Aslan, M et al. "The effect of oxytocin and Kisspeptin-10 in ovary and uterus of ischemia-reperfusion injured rats." *Taiwanese journal of obstetrics & gynecology* 56, no. 4 (August 2017): 456-462. PMID: 28805600. https://doi.org/10.1016/j.tjog.2016.12.018.

119   Seiwerth, Sven et al. "BPC 157 and blood vessels." *Current pharmaceutical design* 20, no. 7 (2014): 1121-5. PMID: 23782145. https://doi.org/10.2174/13816128113199990421.

120   Kutilin, D S, T I Bondarenko, I V Kornienko, and I I Mikhaleva. "Effect of delta sleep-inducing peptide on the expression of antioxidant enzyme genes in the brain and blood of rats during physiological aging." *Bulletin of experimental biology and medicine* 157, no. 5 (September 2014): 616-9. PMID: 25257425. https://doi.org/10.1007/s10517-014-2628-4.

121   Kingsberg, Sheryl A et al. "Bremelanotide for the Treatment of Hypoactive Sexual Desire Disorder: Two Randomized Phase 3 Trials." *Obstetrics and gynecology* 134, no. 5 (November 2019): 899-908. PMID: 31599840. https://doi.org/10.1097/AOG.0000000000003500.

122   Ye, Rui et al. "GHRH expression plasmid improves osteoporosis and skin damage in aged mice." *Growth hormone & IGF research : official journal of the Growth Hormone Research Society and the International IGF Research Society* 60-61 (October-December 2021): 101429. PMID:

34507253. https://doi.org/10.1016/j.ghir.2021.101429; Landin-Wilhelmsen, Kerstin, Anders Nilsson, Inggvar Bosaeus, and Bengt-Ake Bengtsson. "Growth hormone increases bone mineral content in postmenopausal osteoporosis: a randomized placebo-controlled trial." *Journal of bone and mineral research : the official journal of the American Society for Bone and Mineral Research* 18, no. 3 (March 2003): 393-405. PMID: 12619921. https://doi.org/10.1359/jbmr.2003.18.3.393.

123   Sebecić, B et al. "Osteogenic effect of a gastric pentadecapeptide, BPC-157, on the healing of segmental bone defect in rabbits: a comparison with bone marrow and autologous cortical bone implantation." *Bone* 24, no. 3 (March 1999): 195-202. PMID: 10071911. https://doi.org/10.1016/s8756-3282(98)00180-x; Breuil, Véronique et al. "Oxytocin and bone remodelling: relationships with neuropituitary hormones, bone status and body composition." *Joint bone spine* 78, no. 6 (December 2011): 611-5. PMID: 21441053. https://doi.org/10.1016/j.jbspin.2011.02.002; Hu, B-T, and W-Z Chen. "MOTS-c improves osteoporosis by promoting osteogenic differentiation of bone marrow mesenchymal stem cells via TGF-β/Smad pathway." *European review for medical and pharmacological sciences* 22, no. 21 (November 2018): 7156-7163. PMID: 30468456. https://doi.org/10.26355/eurrev_201811_16247.

124   Pickart, Loren, and Anna Margolina. "Regenerative and Protective Actions of the GHK-Cu Peptide in the Light of the New Gene Data." *International journal of molecular sciences* 19, no. 7 (July 2018): 1987. PMID: 29986520. https://doi.org/10.3390/ijms19071987; Pyo, Hyun Keol et al. "The effect of tripeptide-copper complex on human hair growth in vitro." *Archives of pharmacal research* 30, no. 7 (July 2007): 834-9. PMID: 17703734. https://doi.org/10.1007/BF02978833.

125   Gao, Xiao-Yu et al. "Role of thymosin beta 4 in hair growth." *Molecular genetics and genomics : MGG* 291, no. 4 (August 2016): 1639-46. PMID: 27130465. https://doi.org/10.1007/s00438-016-1207-y; Gao, Xiaoyu et al. "Thymosin Beta-4 Induces Mouse Hair Growth." *PloS one* 10, no. 6 (June 2015): e0130040. PMID: 26083021. https://doi.org/10.1371/journal.pone.0130040.

126   Dorr, R T et al. "Evaluation of melanotan-II, a superpotent cyclic melanotropic peptide in a pilot phase-I clinical study." *Life sciences* 58, no. 20 (1996): 1777-84. PMID: 8637402. https://doi.org/10.1016/0024-3205(96)00160-9.

127   Punga, Anna Rostedt, and Maarika Liik. "Botulinum toxin injections associated with suspected myasthenia gravis: An underappreciated cause of MG-like clinical presentation." *Clinical neurophysiology practice* 5 (February 2020): 46-49. PMID: 32140629. https://doi.org/10.1016/j.cnp.2020.01.002.

128   Mehri, Keyvan et al. "Rivastigmine ameliorates botulinum-induced hippocampal damage and spatial memory impairment in male rats." *Neurotoxicology* 98 (September 2023): 29-38. PMID: 37507053. https://doi.org/10.1016/j.neuro.2023.07.004.

www.ingramcontent.com/pod-product-compliance
Lightning Source LLC
LaVergne TN
LVHW012249070526
838201LV00107B/309/J